HOME
SAFE

HOME SAFE

A Memoir of End-of-Life Care
During Covid-19

MITCHELL CONSKY

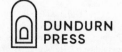

DUNDURN
PRESS

A portion of the royalties from the sale of *Home Safe* will be donated to cancer research at Toronto's Sunnybrook Hospital.

Publisher: Kwame Scott Fraser | Acquiring editor: Julie Mannell | Editor: Dominic Farrell
Cover designer: Laura Boyle | Cover image: istock.com/Dmitriy Maltsev

Library and Archives Canada Cataloguing in Publication

Title: Home safe : a memoir of end-of-life care during Covid-19 / Mitchell Consky.
Names: Consky, Mitchell, author.
Identifiers: Canadiana (print) 20220260036 | Canadiana (ebook) 20220260087 | ISBN 9781459750272 (softcover) | ISBN 9781459750289 (PDF) | ISBN 9781459750296 (EPUB)
Subjects: LCSH: Consky, Mitchell. | LCSH: Fathers—Death. | LCSH: Terminally ill—Home care. | LCSH: Terminal care. | LCSH: COVID-19 Pandemic, 2020-
Classification: LCC R726.8 .C66 2022 | DDC 362.17/5—dc23

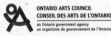

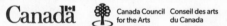

We acknowledge the support of the Canada Council for the Arts and the Ontario Arts Council for our publishing program. We also acknowledge the financial support of the Government of Ontario, through the Ontario Book Publishing Tax Credit and Ontario Creates, and the Government of Canada.

Care has been taken to trace the ownership of copyright material used in this book. The author and the publisher welcome any information enabling them to rectify any references or credits in subsequent editions.

The publisher is not responsible for websites or their content unless they are owned by the publisher.

Printed and bound in Canada.

Dundurn Press
1382 Queen Street East
Toronto, Ontario, Canada M4L 1C9
dundurn.com, @dundurnpress

For Dad and Uncle Norman — our two fallen soldiers who never got the chance to read this, but who encouraged every page.

Other things may change us, but we start and end with family.
— Anthony Brandt

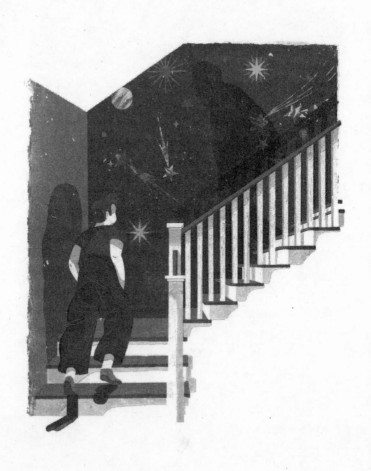

The Top of the Stairs
May 10, 2020[1]

It was almost two in the morning when I entered my parents' house, reeking of marijuana. I disabled the alarm, pulled off my shoes, and sprayed a little Lysol on my sweatshirt. Then I tiptoed out of the laundry room like I always used to when I'd come home late and didn't want to wake anyone from one of the many groaning floorboards.

It all felt so normal — reminding me of those Saturday nights in high school when I'd return from a party, or when I was visiting from university and back from a bar, ready to sleep in my old bed, attempting to slip through the shadows unnoticed.

No matter how sneaky I'd be, though, my father would always greet me at the top of the stairs. Slouching there in his boxers, his eyes groggy, he'd ask me how my night was. I'd ask him why he was up, already knowing the answer — that he

1 Essay originally published in the *Globe and Mail* on June 2, 2020, under the title "Always Watching Over Me" with the illustration (opposite) by Rachel Wada.

could never sleep until he knew I was home safe. No matter how late I came in and no matter how old I got, he needed to check on me and make sure I was okay.

Charley was fast asleep on his mat near the staircase, re-affirming my family's suspicion that he'd make a horrible guard dog. I stroked his curly, white hair and made my way up the stairs, avoiding the creakiest steps, feeling a little guilty that I had been out for so long.

I had been walking around the neighbourhood with my friend Sam, smoking separate joints, keeping six feet apart, and struggling to process my dad's recent diagnosis. I wasn't able to cry during that walk; in fact, I haven't been able to cry for the last couple weeks.

Discovering his Stage 4 cancer was scary enough, but it was even scarier during the onset of a pandemic. All of it was too overwhelming to understand, too heavy to carry. Life throws many curve balls, but rarely with the velocity and frequency of those in the last month; now I was shocked at home plate, feeling as if the universe had struck me out. Maybe what I needed was a hug, one of those big, spine-squeezing embraces, but in a world that required distance, they were no longer available.

His diagnosis came suddenly, a couple weeks after my twenty-fifth birthday, during the infancy of a time when people were afraid to enter a grocery store, let alone an emergency room. Maybe that was the problem. With our biggest fear being the invisible enemy outside, we were blindsided by the one growing inside him.

The result was a switch of roles; when it was typically my father who would check on me, I was now the one checking on him. It was me who would tuck him in at night and make sure he was okay, who would bring him water when he was thirsty, food when he was hungry, morphine to mask his pain, Zofran to ease the nausea. I kept an eye on him around the clock, except for the occasional moment when I slipped away to go on a walk. I was grateful to return the favour, to be there for him the way he'd been there for me my whole life. But as I made it to the top of the stairs that night, I was really hoping I'd see him standing there in his boxers. I was hoping for just one more moment where he was the father and I was the son.

I wasn't surprised that he wasn't there. After his first treatment, he'd been getting weaker and more fatigued. Some days, it was difficult for him to even leave his bed except to go to the bathroom. I had been walking with him down the upstairs hallway once a day to prevent too much atrophy. With my arms prepared to hold him, we'd head toward my bedroom at the end. Sometimes, as he'd make it the whole length, he'd do a little dance, like a football player celebrating a miraculous touchdown, to make my sister and mom laugh, but his pain and exhaustion quickly pulled him back to bed, like it was the final quarter and he had left it all on the field.

After walking down that hallway, I stepped into my childhood room and closed the door softly. My chest shuddered and I suddenly felt cold. I got under the covers, feeling my emotions competing. A part of me worried that I would never have someone who cared for me that way again; a part of me felt thankful that I had someone who cared that way for all those years. Not all sons are so lucky. As I gazed at the dark ceiling, steadying my breathing, I told myself it's not over, that there's still some fight within him. Searching my mind for evidence, I remembered the day my family went hiking in Charlevoix, Quebec, a few summers ago.

Green leaves rustled around us as the four of us trekked through rough terrain. Dad was getting tired; stamina was never his strong suit. He found a bench shaded by pine trees at the halfway point and took a seat. A little too comfy, he insisted we go on without him. But once my mom, my sister, and I made it to the view, overlooking a summit ignited by late-afternoon sunlight, a Gatorade-blue lake glimmering in the distance, we heard the crunching of footsteps and turned to find him tiredly proceeding our way. He never failed to surprise us, mustering strength we never knew he had. I only hoped that strength would return.

A floorboard groaned at the end of the hall, and a bar of light glowed through the bottom of my door. He'd been getting up to pee at least once an hour lately, and my sister, Steph, and I had been alternating each night to check on him. Tonight was her shift, but maybe I'd go anyway. Checking on him when I wasn't on duty would be a small demonstration of the care he always served.

I rolled out of bed, opened my door, and stopped midstep.

There he was, standing before my bedroom in his underwear, about to walk in after making the trip down the hall by himself.

"I just wanted to make sure you were home safe," Dad said, as if nothing had changed in the last month, reminding me that it would take more than cancer to hold him back. That he would always be my father and I would always be his son.

I hugged him tightly, and that coldness I felt was replaced with a familiar warmth.

For the first time in weeks, my eyes began to well.

Part One:
"A Pain in the Ass"

Hemorrhoids
April 9, 2020

A few weeks after the World Health Organization first declared an international health emergency that shut down the planet — causing me to abandon my Toronto apartment to move back into my parents' house — Dad fainted.

It was mid-April, and morning sunlight seeped through my closed shutters. Birds chirped the promise of warmer weather, budding leaves, and that sweet aroma of a long-awaited spring. I just wanted to sleep.

A pillow shielded my eyes, protecting what was previously a peaceful slumber. I rolled over to check my cellphone on my nightstand for the time. It was almost 9:00 a.m. I buried my face under more pillows.

I had been up late the previous night, working on a feature story for the Canadian journalism magazine the *Walrus*, about families of healthcare workers coping with varying degrees of separation during the pandemic. It was going to be my first byline in a national publication, my first big break after my last semester of journalism school.

Hungry to prove my writing chops, I'd been straining over each sentence, lavishing meticulous attention on the few that had been written — a fancy way of saying the words weren't coming despite a fast-approaching deadline. I was exhausted and deflated. And my hope of sleeping in was quickly abandoned when a loud thump rattled my wall.

"Mitchell! Come here! Quick!" My mother's panicked shout jolted me out of bed.

I cannoned down the hall, turned into my parents' bedroom, and halted at the open doorway of their shared bathroom.

Dad was kneeling on the tiled floor in his boxers, next to a small blotch of bright-red blood. "He fainted!" called Mom, standing over him.

"I did not!" Dad called back. He struggled to get back up, but his elbows hit the floor. I looked at the blood on the tile, reflecting the fluorescent lighting of the bathroom. "I just lost my balance a little," he said.

Two days earlier, on the morning of my twenty-fifth birthday, I awoke to find a similar blood spot near the bathroom downstairs. Dad had stubbornly excused the incident as bleeding from an anal fissure, which was caused, he believed, by a bad case of hemorrhoids. That night, another year older and lying in bed restlessly, I did what you should *never* do — I Googled "rectal bleeding from hemorrhoids," and, of course, the worst flashed across my screen.

"By themselves, hemorrhoids are rarely serious, but they can be extremely troublesome. In some instances, they may mask a more serious disorder, such as colon or rectal cancer. Therefore, hemorrhoids require the proper diagnosis and treatment by a physician," one site read. I copied and pasted the warning and texted it to Mom. We chose not to trust Google because — some pun intended here — it's normally just full of shit.

We had been noticing Dad's weight loss but rationalized his lack of appetite with the stress of circumstances: the stock market crashing and an unwillingness to participate in the mass grocery hoarding of a pandemic-panicked society made a few lost pounds understandable.

With all the clinics shut down and Dad unable to receive a physical assessment, he resorted to a virtual meeting with a general surgeon, describing what he was feeling to a laptop screen. It was only a year and a half since he'd had his last colonoscopy, and cancer cells typically take three years to grow. Colon cancer was ruled out, and the symptoms were chalked up to what Dad kept insisting: hemorrhoids. Maybe an anal fissure. But certainly not the big "C." Definitely not an anorectal melanoma tumour that had spread to his liver, lymph nodes, and lungs. That would be extremely unlikely, and, given the brand-new pandemic, *the worst fucking timing ever.*

But after finding him on the floor, we knew the problem couldn't be ignored. Fortunately, we had more than a few numbers to call.

Most of my extended family work in healthcare. Our roster of siblings, aunts, uncles, and cousins includes three emergency physicians, a neurologist, two social workers, a nurse, and a registered dietitian who's dating, and lives with, a general surgery resident. Normally, having a team of healthcare professionals in your family is merely advantageous. It can save you a trip to the doctor's office, dismantle medical anxieties (a symptom of too many Google searches), and help lift the haze of medical jargon that shrouds patients far and wide. But whatever benefits we were accustomed to accessing had evaporated in the time of Covid-19. The immediate medical support we once had was unavailable; our soldiers were now fighting another war, too deep in the trenches to help with the personal one not yet declared. But we knew they'd answer their phones.

Mom called her brother, Norman — one of the three emergency physicians in the family. I called my cousin Daniel and Uncle Howie — the two others. We also called my sister, Steph, a registered dietitian, who was with her boyfriend, Ryan, the general surgery resident.

After we merged calls, our conversations were sporadic and short. They fired a whirlwind of questions, and we answered what we could.

"What's his pulse?"

"What's his heart rate?"

"Does he have a fever?"

"How long has he had these symptoms?"

"What colour is his urine?"

"How much blood is there?"

"Just a little, like a tablespoon …" I said, pacing.

"A tablespoon of blood would look like a murder scene; it always looks like more. So, it's probably less. What colour is it?"

"Bright red …"

"Any other symptoms now?"

"He's short of breath, having difficulty — Dad, sit down! — keeping upright — Dad, stop looking for your phone! — and he's as distracted as normal."

Finally, after enough context was provided, Daniel told me what I feared: "Look, Mitch … I think you should take him to the Emerg."

Daniel was one of the ER doctors I had interviewed for the *Walrus* story about healthcare workers. A week prior he told me about the panicked state of the emergency department, how physicians are almost exclusively treating patients in critical condition. I knew he wouldn't tell us to go unless he thought it was absolutely necessary.

Maybe it was clear that we should've taken him the second we found him on the floor — any other time we would've put him in the car the second we suspected something was wrong. But in those early weeks of the pandemic, when most people were afraid to walk out their front door, widely uncertain as to what that invisible enemy was, the thought of sending Dad into a hospital filled me with a new type of horror.

"Okay," I said.

"And Mitch," Daniel added before I hung up.

"Yeah?"

He gave me advice that was not yet widely recommended by health experts for the general public, advice, in early April 2020, ascribed exclusively to patients in healthcare facilities.

"Bring a mask," he said. "All of you."

Behind the Glass
September 7, 2017

An old marquee sign, with bulbs no longer functional, showed what was playing: *Despicable Me 3*. Tickets were nine bucks for adults and seniors — seven for children. The evening show started at eight, but it was closer to eight twenty when we walked through the front doors into the aroma of freshly popped popcorn.

Movie posters decorated the red walls — there was a faded one for *Rocky II*, with a beaten Sylvester Stallone in a boxing stance, struggling to stay upright, his eyes swollen, his red gloves glowing in the grainy spotlight. To the left of the snack bar was a crowded display of rusted projector equipment and, in a shadowed hall, a glass cabinet filled with dusty film reels.

Dad peered at the items showcased like ancient fossils in a museum.

"Show's already started," said a woman in an apron behind us. "Still want tickets?" She was sweeping some scattered popcorn into a dustpan coated with pieces of chewed gum. The muffled speakers of the auditorium behind buzzed softly.

I looked over at Dad. He seemed tired, distracted.

"No thanks," I said.

"Well, can I help you?"

"My grandparents built this theatre," I said, with a note of pride. I patted Dad on his shoulder. "His parents ... He grew up here."

"Welcome back," she said to him, smiling wide. "Are you two just visiting for the weekend?"

Dad didn't respond, so I did. "Yeah ... We came from Toronto. Wanted a father and son road trip before I go back to school in a week."

"Ah, that's nice."

Kernels started crackling out of the bowl of the popcorn machine.

"Do you guys still use coconut oil and Savoral on the kernels?" Dad asked. Savoral is a seasoning salt he often raved about; it gives the popcorn a synthetic buttery taste that competing flavour chemicals can't quite match. (Anyone who says they prefer natural ingredients in their popcorn is a liar.)

"Don't think we do," she said.

Dad nodded. It was another small reminder of how much had changed. His eyes fell back to the glass case.

✳

Visiting his hometown offered a keyhole-look into an innocent past now locked away. His memories were invaded by a
changing landscape — cut-down trees, ripped-down buildings, fewer shops, and fewer people. It was a town both familiar and alien, incompatible with the warm glow of nostalgia
that pulled him back in the first place.

Mattawa is an Algonquin term for "meeting of waters."
The sleepy town in northeastern Ontario, dwarfed by looming
hills of dense greenery, sits at the confluence of the Mattawa
and Ottawa rivers in the Nipissing District, half an hour's drive
east from North Bay. When he lived there in the fifties and six-
ties, for the first fourteen years of his life, Dad felt connected
to a vibrant community of working-class families — friendly
faces, barking dogs, laughing kids. It was like any other small
town, with fishing derbies and town hall meetings and local
gossip about who did what. But it now seemed smaller.

"It's strange how different it all feels," he said as we arrived
after the four-hour drive north from Toronto, with "Happiness
Is a Warm Gun" playing on the radio. We had found a station that was featuring the top hundred Beatles songs, and the
timeless hits made the car ride seem shorter.

Eventually, we checked into a motel that he remembered as
the local "standard of reliable comfort" but now had mildew
on the walls.

Later that evening, as we walked down narrow sidewalks,
he pointed out what he remembered, and ignored what he

didn't. Across the road from where his school used to be was his old family house, the one his parents designed and built — no longer nestled by trees. He showed me the backyard where his father built an ice rink, the door where his mother used to call him and his siblings in for dinner, and the bedroom window he used to look out from, the one facing the backyard that opened up toward Main Street.

❋

The four-hundred-and-twenty-two-seat movie theatre his parents operated, with its two-hundred-inch screen and fully equipped snack bar, was a short walk through the backyard gate, down a narrow path, and across the road.

"We've improved our projector system since those days," said the woman, gesturing to the rusted equipment on display. "Everything's digital now. We also upgraded the sound system. Would you like to see the new projector room?"

Dad's parents died when he was young — his mother when he was fourteen, his father when he was twenty-two. He rarely spoke about them. The movie theatre stood as a lasting reminder of his parents and of the life he once lived, a lingering projection of images too pixelated to fully recall. Maybe it bothered him to see his parents' equipment now obsolete. Maybe it reminded him of life's impermanence, of how things kept on flowing, of the future that had washed away the past like the Mattawa and Ottawa rivers merging in rapid flux.

"No thanks," Dad said to the woman. "Mitch, let's get going."

I waved goodbye and followed him back onto the dark road. The clouds had cleared, leaving a purple sky; pink streaks edged over the horizon. "Dad, why didn't you want to see it?" I asked as we made it to the car. I knew it hurt him, but I wanted him to talk about it.

"We'll look at it next time," he said, climbing inside.

Knowing "next time" wouldn't be anytime soon, I opened the door and looked back at the old theatre once more.

I had heard snippets about his life growing up there — racing his brother, Earl, through the aisles; calling his food order to his sister, Louise, who sometimes helped at the snack bar ("Popcorn, hotdog, a Virginia bar, and a Coke, please!"); watching new releases as their parents worked nearby …

Dad was a successful Toronto lawyer now, operating his own firm, and his life in Mattawa was far behind him. There was so much he never spoke about, so much he locked away and kept beyond reach, like the dusty film reels behind glass.

I think it hurt him to bring up the idyllic childhood that lay beyond reach, the loss of security that plagued his past with the absence of his mother's affection, the empty void in any man cut off from fatherly guidance too young.

Mostly, though, I think it reminded him of what was impossible to avoid no matter how fast he drove away: every good film, regardless of how beautiful it may be, comes to an end.

The engine rattled to life, and Dad hit the gas.

Two Masks
April 2020

Our car rolled into the parking lot of the North York General Hospital's emergency department. There was a tunnel outside the entrance covered in tight black plastic. Three security guards stood at the front of it, wearing face masks and plastic face shields.

We wondered if there was a separate entrance for patients without Covid symptoms. I got out of the car to ask one of the security guards. The moment I approached, one of them took a step back.

"Is there a separate line for non-Covid patients?" I called through my mask, standing a good distance away.

"All emergency patients go through here," one called back. "Only the patient is allowed in."

I went back into the car. "Dad, you need to go through that tunnel," I said. "They won't let anyone else come with you."

He nodded, and I squirted some hand sanitizer into his hands. I gave him the mini-bottle, and he slid it into his pocket.

"Don't touch anything," called Mom in the driver's seat. "Especially not your face."

"Why not?" Dad said, playing dumb.

The whole ride up he had been cracking lame jokes to calm us down. Things like, "Look ... whatever this is ... at least I still have two arms," referring to the one-armed zookeeper in

Tiger King, the Netflix docuseries we binge-watched days before. Then … "*Oh fuck*, a tiger!" he called, thrashing around in his seat with a reusable grocery bag on his arm.

"Cut it out, Harvey!" Mom barked. "I'm driving!"

Boyish humour had long been his way of coping with stress, and a method for easing the anxieties of those around him. He was wearing two masks — one to protect him from the virus, and one to protect us from worrying. One wasn't on properly — I adjusted the elastic over his ear after we got out of the car. The other was ineffective.

"Trump says the virus is a hoax," he added. "Why would he lie? He seems like a real straight shooter!"

"Not funny, Harv," Mom called with an eye roll.

And it wasn't. On this day, New York state would confirm its highest daily total of first-wave fatalities: 1,028 people would die from complications related to the coronavirus in that state alone. The numbers coming out of Europe were even worse. In Toronto, the epicentre for the SARS epidemic, we were desperately hoping we wouldn't follow suit.

Dad's glasses fogged up a little, and the two of us walked toward the entrance as Mom waited in the car. It was a blue-sky morning, and sunlight beamed down on us.

"I love you, Dad," I said.

"I love you more," he replied. "And don't argue." That's what he always said to my mom, sister, and me. He loved us more, and that was final.

For a moment, those hazel eyes behind his foggy lenses made him look younger than the sixty-seven-year-old he was.

There was a furrow in his brow, a tightness in his jaw, but his cheeks forced a smile beneath the fabric covering his mouth — he was adjusting his other mask. "I'll be okay," he said.

"I know you will … No tigers in there."

Dad nodded. Then he walked through that black tunnel alone.

Hit by a Car
May 6, 1963

"Harvey was hit by a car!"

The words rattled through Earl's mind as he sprinted down Main Street, toward the hospital on the other side of the bridge. His breathing was harsh as his sneakers pounded concrete.

Louise trailed closely, but he was gaining distance. His sister was a year older, but Earl's legs gave him a longer stride. He was almost thirteen, and his shoe size was the same number. Nearly five foot nine, he towered over Harvey, who was only a year younger but hardly cleared five foot one — a more common height for a boy his age. Earl's chest tightened as he crossed the bridge and saw the town hospital in the distance.

He was in the ticket office, around 3:00 p.m., when the phone rang and Louise answered. Her face went pale as a voice told her what happened — her little brother, who had been off on a bike ride near Champlain Provincial Park fifteen minutes outside of town, had been hit by a car. He was in the hospital.

She shouted what she'd learned to Earl, and the two siblings sprinted out the movie theatre's front door into the cool May air. The hospital was only ten minutes from the theatre, but it felt like a marathon away.

Apart from her birth, Louise had never been inside that hospital. Earl was born there, too. Harvey's claim to fame was that he, the youngest of the trio, was born half an hour outside of town, in the "big city" of North Bay.

They turned a corner and found the room.

Their little brother was sitting upright on the hospital bed. Aside from gauze wrapped around the left side of his head, where he had recently received fourteen stitches, he looked like himself. Louise detected her little brother's fear, though. Harvey was eleven, but, sitting there between his parents, he appeared so much younger. He was a child who had never known real danger before.

Neither had his siblings. In their safe, small-town life, this was the first time anything had gone seriously wrong. They weren't isolated from distant tragedies — there had been the death of an uncle from cancer, the heart attack that ended the life of the grandfather they never knew, those peripheral understandings of grief and loss. But never had they been confronted with the fragility of their own young existence.

Harvey didn't remember much of what had happened. He was pedalling along the country road, feeling the May breeze on his face, when he heard the roar of an engine. A swerving flash caught the corner of his eye, and before he could jolt his handlebars, the car hit him and launched him off his seat.

He found himself on the grass, staring at the blurry sky. Whoever hit him didn't stop.

He remembered feeling some blood. The next thing he was able to recall was being in the hospital with his parents. His mother's caring eyes put him at ease.

Her eyes were big and brown, glimmering with the compassion and empathy that can be found in the gaze of any mother who shows endless love to her children. His father, standing by her side, conveyed a calming warmth, lending a presence that could dial down the anxiety of those around him.

When his brother and sister walked into that hospital wing, though, the fear that still showed on Harvey's face disappeared. He saw their concern, and he put on a forced smile that masked his own. "I'm okay," he said.

Earl and Louise hugged him tightly.

"Really. I'm okay," he repeated, wrapped in his siblings' arms.

They embraced. Their parents comforted them, and the familiar feeling of security returned. Life would continue as normal. No consequences would catch up with the reckless driver who almost killed a kid. No lasting injuries would remain.

More than fifty years later, the memory, as ultimately inconsequential as it was, would be one of the most specifically detailed events of my aunt, uncle, and father's past. Many childhood memories would fade or become disjointed and foggy and difficult to articulate precisely. But, for all three of them, that day would remain clear.

I think it's because the memory carries a lesson, one known subconsciously or consciously, a clichéd one, maybe, but one that rings important and true: life can change in an instant.

And for my family, it was about to.

Lucky
April 15, 2020

I heard her words, but their meaning didn't register. Standing barefoot on the basement carpet, holding my cellphone against my ear, I gazed at a shelf of family photos.

One stand-up frame held an image of Steph and me — her as a pig-tailed, smiling toddler; me as a dazed, seemingly constipated infant. Another had an image of Steph, age five or six, with Mom and Dad. She's sitting on Dad's lap after a dance recital, hugging a bundle of roses.

To the right of it was another photo, of the four of us on vacation somewhere. My eyes focused on Dad's gentle face, his squinty smile, dark eyebrows, receding hairline. "I don't know what you're saying," I said, breathing a little quicker, desperate to awake from the nightmare — for the pandemic to end, for my family to unite in one physical space, for the tumour to be benign. Steph was telling me the last of those was unlikely.

She was saying that all his symptoms aligned with the word nobody was willing to say, the one all of us couldn't stop thinking about. "We can only hope it didn't spread," she said. Then, "I love you, Mitch. I wish I could be with you."

But she couldn't. Steph worked as a registered dietitian at a long-term care home for seniors, and her floor had recently had an outbreak; a growing number of the staff were infected with the virus. She was awaiting her own test results, uncertain as to when she would be able to come home. She didn't want to risk Dad getting sicker than he already was — how sick he was we didn't yet know.

"I love you, too," I said. Steph's voice was comforting, but, in that moment, what we both needed was a hug — a physical embrace, like a pinch, that would confirm we weren't dreaming.

The call ended, and I broke my gaze from the shelf of photos. Sobbing, I collapsed onto the floor.

❦

After some examinations at North York General, an ER physician ordered an emergency colonoscopy to get a biopsy on a mass they found growing on Dad's rectum. They didn't know what it was, but it was ulcerated — the cause of the bleeding — and definitely not hemorrhoids. The doctor also arranged a CT scan.

If it weren't for Dad collapsing on the bathroom floor, the threat might've continued unnoticed. A couple of extra-strength Advils he had swallowed to numb the pain that morning had thinned his blood enough to cause severe bleeding. ("It'd make a great Advil commercial," Dad later joked.)

He endured further examinations with a positive attitude, always being sure to express his gratitude to every doctor, nurse, and technician who helped the process. "Thank you very much," he'd say. "I'm lucky to have your help." He used the word *lucky* strangely often for someone in his circumstances.

But as we waited for the results, we weren't sure how lucky he was. He was definitely thinner than he'd ever been; the roundness in his face had deflated slightly — his cheekbones were suddenly more pronounced. Yet, in an unexpected way, he also glowed.

His hair had grown out because he hadn't been able to visit his shut-down barbershop, and there was a light stubble on his cheeks. He looked energetic, healthy. A couple of days after he returned from the hospital, I caught him flexing shirtless in front of a mirror, like an adolescent boy examining his changing body. He had always had a gut that he was trying to burn off, but he was now as slim as he was when he was my age. There was jarring irony in knowing how sick he might have been and seeing how healthy he appeared. A part of me believed he was okay. That he was better than ever.

But four days after his colonoscopy and two days after his CT scan, he got the call.

"Uh-huh … Uh-huh …" Dad was pacing in the living room with his cellphone pressed against his ear.

"Dad! Put it on speaker!" I shouted.

He waved his hand in front of my face. "Uh-huh ... I see ... Okay ..."

Mom walked into the kitchen. "Is that —"

"Yes! And he won't put him on speaker!"

"Harvey, put it on speaker!" Mom hissed.

"Okay, Doctor ... Uh-huh." That's when his face changed. His eyes widened slightly, and he dropped onto the couch in the family room. "It's some type of melanoma," Dad said to us, still listening.

I ripped the phone out of his hand and hit the speaker icon. "— 90 percent certain it spread to your liver," we heard.

"Oh my God," Mom muttered.

"I've arranged for more tests, but I also set up an appointment for you to meet with Dr. Petrella at Sunnybrook. She's one of the top melanoma specialists in the country."

"Thank you very much, Doctor," Dad said. "I'm lucky to have your help."

Shortly after, he hung up.

At first, I felt absolutely nothing. Complete emptiness had expanded inside me as I remained on my knees on the living-room carpet. But then I saw the tears in Dad's eyes, then Mom's, and next thing I knew I was burying my face in Dad's chest like a small child.

He always used to tell me I would sleep on his chest when I was a baby. I'm pretty sure all babies do that, but he would tell me this like it was special to me, like it was a unique bond only we shared. At that moment, I wished I was a baby again. I wished I could lie on his chest and feel his belly rising and falling, certain that another breath would come, that the pumping heart I'm connected to would continue pumping, that life wouldn't so soon slip away.

Mom cried into his shoulder. I squeezed her hand. Dad squeezed mine. Charley started barking. We all held each other, and, feeling the incompleteness of our family unit, I wished Steph was with us. I wished all four of us were home safe.

"We'll do our best to beat this," Dad said eventually. He gulped, like he was swallowing his disbelief. "I'm lucky we're getting help so fast."

There was that word again.

He stood up and walked to the next room, his posture slightly more erect, with the look of concentration on his face he often had when he was working out a case in his mind, or before he was about to enter a courtroom, wearing a robe, holding a briefcase. Dad's life had been full of tremendous challenges, and now there was one more, one big one, that would suddenly make all the others seem small.

He didn't look defeated. His chin was up. His eyes were now dry. It was as if he had allowed himself a moment of weakness but then decided it was time to move on and get to business.

Lucky. The word repeated in my mind. How could he possibly feel *lucky*?

The Bed
April 16, 2020

With tears on Stephanie's cheeks beginning to dry, she paced around her condo living room and tried to devise a plan that would make it possible for her to give her father a hug. With a long exhale, she realized a difficult decision had to be made.

Steph thought back to the chain of emails she had received from the management of the long-term care home she worked at, informing her that five staff members on her floor had recently tested positive for the virus. There were three infected at the end of March and two more by the middle of April. The emails nudged employees to stay home if they, or anyone near them, were showing any signs of symptoms. But they also expressed the urgent need for all employees to report for duty if they were healthy. There were vulnerable seniors that needed protection, and every healthcare facility needed all sanitized hands on deck.

Wind howled against the large windowpanes behind the couch, and Steph stopped pacing to gaze at the concrete jungle beyond the foggy glass. In pre-pandemic times, the nighttime cityscape would sparkle with the lights of passing cars, glowing storefronts, and the fluorescent mosaic of office buildings illuminating the skyline. It still glowed and glimmered, but, tonight, Toronto shone a little less brightly.

Steph wondered how many others out there felt so isolated and afraid. A part of her wanted to go back in time, to the days, just a few weeks earlier, when those chaotic streets were congested with streams of rushing civilians. Another part of her wanted to speed time up a week. That's how long it would take to determine if it was safe for her to go back home, to be near family.

But the thing was ... she wouldn't know *for sure* if it was safe. Not really. There was always the possibility of a false negative, especially with those early testing kits. What if she was asymptomatic? Or what if the symptoms were only now emerging?

She pushed the thought away, knowing the paranoia was just as contagious as the virus itself. Covid wasn't her top concern — it was far down her list now. But, along with changing everything around her, it stood as a barrier between her and her sick father, one she did not yet know how to manoeuvre.

As she collapsed onto the couch, her breathing began to quicken again. Her eyes fell on the coffee table, that thousand-piece jigsaw puzzle of a pug's wrinkled face, which she had spent hours piecing together when time hadn't seemed so limited. Next to it was the photo book she had designed and printed, featuring shots from a recent trip to Colombia she had taken with her boyfriend, Ryan.

Tonight, Ryan was on call at a Toronto hospital where three staff members had tested positive the previous week. Each night Ryan came home and threw his scrubs in the wash, the risk of exposure was reintroduced.

Steph missed Ryan. She thought about how she had met him on that Tinder date three years before, at the wine-tasting restaurant he suggested downtown. He was just beginning his general surgery residency then. She had just wrapped up her nutrition and dietetics training and was in the process of submitting job applications to clinics and hospitals.

She remembered first seeing his full moustache — it was like a cop's in an eighties crime drama. He told her he'd never shave it because of some long-standing bet with one of his med-school buddies. Steph got used to it and would eventually enjoy the conspiratorial chatter of her cousins jokingly plotting to shave it off in his sleep.

His sensitive side came out with his passion for jazz, a love for plants, and the poems he wrote on birthday cards for Steph when they first started dating. "When I'm with you, life slows down for a while.… Happy birthday to the girl with the brightest smile," one went. After she first learned something was wrong with Dad, Ryan stayed up with her all night and comforted her as she cried.

Steph knew self-isolating was impossible with the continuous exposure that was a result of living with Ryan. The World Health Organization had speculated that the virus lingered on surfaces, although they were uncertain for how long. (At this point, we were hardly sure if the virus was an aerosol or not.) For all she knew, it was on her couch.

Steph shot up and began to pace again. When she was growing up, Dad would always calm her down when her stress was overwhelming. Whenever she'd call home, he'd answer with a cheerful, "Consky Kennels! No dog too big, no dog too small! We take them all!" (It was a joke he stuck to since we first brought our dog Charley home ten years prior.) On nights she felt overwhelmed or anxious or afraid, he'd offer to pick her up — no matter how far away she was — and he'd take her on a long car ride, sometimes imparting words of support, sometimes saying nothing, with the radio filling the silence. The car humming along the dark road and Dad gripping the steering wheel by her side would somehow make all her tension dissipate. Now she only hoped he had a fighting chance to drive her yet again.

Ryan had helped speed up the process of receiving the biopsy results from the emergency colonoscopy. He had emailed one of his former general surgery supervisors who happened to be overseeing the case, writing that the patient named Harvey Consky was his "father-in-law," because it sounded better than "girlfriend's dad."

"Make good on that promise," Dad had said after Ryan told him this on the phone, causing some nervous laughter. They'd been dating for three years and living together for one. But things had become … challenging.

Despite sharing a living space, they didn't see each other often, even before the pandemic. Over the last two months, most of their time together was spent sleeping in the same bed, which was disrupted by Ryan rising early, chugging a peanut-butter-loaded smoothie, and heading out the door in scrubs by five in the morning. He often didn't return from his shift until Steph was half-asleep the following night.

Busy with her own career, she never complained about his demanding schedule, understanding that the beast of general surgery residency was simply impossible to tame. She knew how solid their relationship was, how distance wouldn't lessen their closeness, but if she had to leave the condo for a period to be with Dad, the little time they had together would suddenly shrink to even less. Not only did she have to face this dilemma, she also had to shoulder her responsibility to report to duty as a healthcare worker, her obligation to help her senior patients in this critical moment in history. Her life, in short, was pulling her in too many directions.

There were words her father once told her that illuminated this struggle — words, weeks later, she would cling on to. *Life is a series of compromises.*

Steph knew where she needed to go.

Invincible
April 17, 2020

The showerhead spat warm water over my face, and steam filled the bathroom. Three short sentences cycled through my mind: Dad has cancer. Steph can't come home. The world has shut down.

Lathering liquid soap over my body, I reminded myself that *I* wasn't dying. Whatever happened, *my* life would some- how continue. But that was hard to believe when everything had completely stopped.

The timing of this was almost comical: normally, when some- one receives such a grave diagnosis, they ignorantly — almost selfishly — expect the world to halt in its tracks, for a quiet stillness to fill the air, underscoring the fact that nothing will ever be the same. And, typically, the world keeps orbiting exactly as it did before. Life continues as it always does — a fast-tracked routine of honking cars and revolving doors that stops for no one. With my dad's diagnosis, however, the world did stop. For *everyone*. His illness may not have been the cause, but it felt as if it was.

The looming uncertainty, the fear that the "normal" lives we had led were now beyond reach, and the horror of a dire future hurtling our way — like a train on tracks we'd been tied to — now seemed the shared state of everyone. It made it difficult to breathe. How long until impact? I imagined my father tied to those tracks, alone, and me standing far away, wanting desperately to move him. But not being able to. I was paralyzed, immobile, helpless. The tracks were vibrating, pistons screaming, engine steaming … *Pst-Pst-Pst-Pst!*

As water sprayed against my back, I wondered how many sons were feeling the same fear right now. How many daughters, or wives, or grandchildren had to face losing a loved one? How many of them had to stand helplessly separated?

Well … I might've been helpless, but I wasn't looking from afar. In a way, my father was fortunate — he had a different disease. He wasn't heaving on a ventilator. He wasn't isolated in a hospital wing with no one around him but masked nurses attending his every breath. We didn't know how long he had — in fact, we didn't know much at all — but we knew we could hold his hand. And knowing that somehow made it all a little less of a nightmare. I wondered if he felt that, too.

I rubbed shampoo on my scalp, trying to calm my buzzing brain. But my mind swerved through lanes of memory, roaring like a speeding motorcycle, driving me to another night, a distant time, five years before a deadly virus brought the world to its knees. It was December 2, 2015, shortly before midnight, when I was first confronted with the fragility of life. Similarly, I was standing in the shower.

❖

The pressure on that showerhead was weak, and the water splattered more than sprayed. It was my third year of university, when I was twenty and invincible. Rinsing foam off my arms, I heard a knock on my bathroom door.

"What's up?"

"Where's your phone?" called my roommate.

"Dead." I had been working late at the student newspaper office, a crowded space where computers shut down spontaneously and electrical outlets were notoriously unreliable.

He walked in, and I opened the shower's flimsy plastic door. His face was ghost-pale in the rising steam. His eyes were wide and bloodshot.

"What's wrong?"

"Gaby Barsky," he said, struggling to summon the next words, "got into a motorcycle accident and ... passed away."

Passed away?

It was a phrase you'd use for an old man — for a grand-parent who had lived a full life. Not someone my age. Not a kid. Not *Gaby*.

Gaby was my fraternity brother. We grew up in the same town, went to the same high school, were counsellors at the same summer camp — we lived similar lives. He was good with computer code. I was good with words. He liked vodka. I liked rum. He was living in California for a co-op term, working for a sports-tech company. I took on a job as opinion editor of the student paper. His recent pay cheques afforded him a motorbike. My recent honorarium covered a couple of pizzas. Discrepancies aside, a thirst for adventure was the common denominator in our friendship.

We once cliff jumped together across the lake from our summer camp — literally linked arms — and our bodies hit the water at different times thanks to an untimed surrender to gravity; an elbow hit my jaw, a head hit my head, a leg hit my groin; hitting the water felt like slamming into concrete. Needless to say, it hurt like a bitch.

We laughed about it as we treaded water, gasping in pain and humour. It was another fun adventure, another cool moment that celebrated our invincibility. We had our fair share of those.

In those college days, we'd streak any time, any place — our clothes would be flying behind us as we'd take off into the winter night, or at venues where alcohol was served a little too cheap. Gaby once tried teaching me to do a backflip. (I hurt my head then, too.) He once yanked a snapping turtle out of the water by the tail, that summer we painted ourselves yellow, pretending to be "Golden Snitches" for our campers who would try to tackle us with hockey sticks between their legs. Together, we talked about the rush of going skydiving, of feeling the still world beneath us as if we're floating, flying like superheroes. We carried youthful ignorance with heads held high, believing that nothing could stop us. Believing that mistakes could be made, lessons learned, and that time was as bottomless as the beer that we poured endlessly into our red Solo cups.

But as I stepped out of the shower that December night, with all my week's problems washing down the drain, it seemed like all time had been cut off, like we'd missed the last call of invincibility. From then on, it no longer mattered if you were young and wild. It no longer mattered if you had nothing but open roads before you. All it took was the vroom of a bike and a car changing lanes to end it all.

A bunch of us cried into each other's shoulders at the frat house that night. We hugged the shit out of each other. Patted backs and kissed heads. We sat there in that dingy, beer-reeking living room, crying an endless mantra of *I love you, man*. It was as if we were trying to remind each other that we were not alone in our confusion. That *we* were still there, and life would somehow continue forward. I didn't know how.

I went on a walk a little later, alone, wandering through empty streets around four in the morning. The stillness was overwhelming, taunting. The only sound was the drum of my feet on concrete, the silence-cutting crunch of dried leaves under my boots. Red Solo cups littered the sidewalk. Shattered beer bottles were scattered over the lawns. Lost in what was once an oasis of celebration, the quietness of the party coming to an end had never felt so final.

My biggest fear had always been that I would leave this world misunderstood, that when I die all my thoughts and memories would die with me. But the strongest reassurance I always had was that words don't die. Words are the only anchor we have; they secure our existence, preventing us from drifting away. They ensure that the party never ends.

I went back to my dorm and wrote Gaby's obituary that night. As the early morning sunlight ignited the new day, I pounded letters on my keyboard at the pace of my pumping heart. I articulated my confusion, my anger, my heartbreak, and I tried to capture his essence, knowing I'd fall short.

I knew that news of Gaby's death was going to break soon, and I needed everyone to know that his life was more than the road accident that ended it. More than a tragic headline. I wrote about his big-tooth smile, his compassionate soul, his computer-nerd demeanour enhanced by a party-boy lovability. I wrote about his love of dancing.

I searched for some takeaway from this loss, some lesson to suggest meaning in the meaningless. "We must not be afraid," I wrote. "But we must not live completely fearless. We must know we are not invincible." The piece was published on the student newspaper site the next day. A storm of heart emojis, like buttons, and "RIP Gaby Barsky" posts later, life moved on — that stream of normality pulled everyone forward — but I didn't.

✦

Gaby had a twin sister, Sabrina. At the funeral, standing before her brother's grave on a cold winter's day, she read out a poem Gaby had written in elementary school on yin and yang, the ancient Chinese philosophy about how the dualism of opposite forces creates harmony in the world. The poem said his sister was yin, like the moon in darkness, and he was yang, the sun shining brightly. He wrote that the two forces balanced each other. That they needed one another to illuminate their way.

Seeing her tear-filled eyes, which so closely resembled those of my good friend, I knew I needed to find some sunshine. Some trace of his warmth and presence. In any small way, I needed to bring him back.

Words were my tools of resurrection. Every night I wrote Sabrina a different memory of growing up with Gaby and sent it to her at 3:00 a.m. (I don't think sleeping was a recognized concept back then.) They were stupid little stories, wildly insignificant, chronicling moments like getting into our first bar with fake IDs and getting kicked out immediately after because Gaby asked for a Molson Canadian in the most nervous voice possible, prompting the bartender to take another look at our cards. Or that time we danced on stage at a sorority fundraiser to "Hakuna Matata," which abruptly escalated to a *Magic Mike* striptease to "It's Raining Men." (We were kicked out of there, too.) For each story, I crafted funny titles, included photos, interviewed witnesses.

Sabrina woke up each morning and laughed about some dumb thing her brother did, and I went to sleep each night exhausted by the battle of immortalization.

Months passed, and eventually my own stories were running low. I reached out to Gaby's friends and asked if they had any anecdotes they'd be willing to share. I scheduled different stories for different nights. I made a Gmail account and hustled people I didn't even know to submit something, anything, that could keep Sabrina's twin alive.

The stories kept rolling. Gaby at a music festival. Gaby's first kiss. Gaby making snow angels under a streetlight on a white-powdered road. I was an intrepid reporter, the editor of a publication that catered content to a one-person audience, content that was also *about* one person. Sabrina got used to receiving the recounts, and I got used to scavenging for them. She told me often how much she appreciated them, how the stories — if only momentarily — illuminated some of the darkness. It was the most important job of my life, but I wasn't only doing it for her.

Sometimes distant friends had a good Gaby moment lingering in the crannies of their memory, but they didn't trust their ability to adequately put it into words. I threw on my journalist hat — a hat I wasn't sure fit yet — and wrote it for them. I interviewed people outside of clubs, and in the smoking pit outside of bars, holding my iPhone to their face with coils of tobacco smoke wafting around me, sometimes with rain splattering against gutters. I pressed for any detail that could enrich the tale, turn the foggy recollection into a memory, a memory into an anecdote, an anecdote into a story. Because the stories were all he left behind. And I made it my mission to collect every last one of them. I did this because I was afraid of him being forgotten. Forgotten by others. Forgotten by me.

Eight months passed, and I had sent Sabrina more than 240 stories. It felt good to have them all written, accessible whenever I needed to remind myself of those younger days when anything seemed possible. But there was so much I never asked him, so much I wish I knew about him before his life was so suddenly wasted. What would Gaby have told the world if he knew he was going to die? What message, what lesson, would've come from the kid taken too soon?

I had dreams about interviewing him, the same way I interviewed his many friends to get the details of a funny story. I dreamed of going back in time, slowing everything down, and asking him any question I could think of. I fantasized about recording them and having not only his words, but also his voice, saved and captured forever. I knew that these fantasies could never have materialized unless Gaby knew he was going to die, or at least considered the imminent possibility. Such considerations do not surface in the minds of the invincible.

❋

As death literature often suggests, denial of our mortality can prevent us from saying what's really on our mind, what we're really feeling, what we really fear, what we really hope for, what keeps us going in times of darkness. Gaby didn't have the chance to express his deepest vulnerabilities.

But my father would.

There was so much Dad kept buried. The pain of losing his mother a year after moving to a big city. Then losing his father seven years later. What it felt like to live parentless in his twenties, supported by the devotion of his brother and sister. The moments of sadness and love that helped shape who he was.

With warm water streaming over my goosebumped skin, I realized I couldn't cure his cancer, but I could learn his story. I can interview him every day and capture his voice and words forever.

I got out of the shower, dried off, and looked over at my iPhone on the counter next to the sink. My family of health-care workers had been bombarding us with information about his prognosis, about clinical trials, about the potential success of certain treatments, recommended medications, even sent reviews of his oncology specialist at Sunnybrook. I knew they'd do whatever it took to prolong his life, to give him a fighting chance.

But my role, besides helping in any way I could, would be different, more symbolic, maybe. Because no matter what happened, I'd keep my father alive.

Oxygen Mask
April 18, 2020

CNN's Anderson Cooper was talking about patients hooked up to ventilators as my mother, Arlene, gazed vacantly at the bedroom television, emotional numbness mingling with physical exhaustion. Harvey was sleeping in the spare bedroom across the hall, which was closer to the bathroom. A light snore — amplified by his CPAP machine — was barely audible beneath the droning TV.

Arlene hugged a pillow, breathing slowly, her bloodshot eyes glued to the screen. Processing her husband's diagnosis was draining, to say the least, and the evening news — as fear mongering as it was — offered brief distraction. But no distraction could drain the flood of fear welling up inside her. She knew what could lie ahead. A memory glimmered.

"I just want to emphasize that nobody needs to talk if they don't feel comfortable." About eight people, men and women in their seventies and eighties, sat around a large table with a pitcher of water and a stack of plastic cups. Daylight filtered into the hospital room. The memory was specific, but it was no different from the countless other sessions Arlene had facilitated.

"Caregiving is a challenging job," Arlene said gently. "But I think you'll find that sharing your experience and listening to the difficulties of others might make you feel less alone."

Arlene is a social worker at the same senior health centre as Steph. She counsels the caregivers of those in need of full-time care, supporting families that have to watch their loved ones progressively decline.

The group consisted of spouses who were in the beginning-to-end stages of caregiving. One woman, whose husband had late-stage dementia, spoke eloquently. "Few things are more difficult to watch than seeing the person you spent your life with wither away," she said, after explaining the gruelling task of changing her husband's adult diapers. "But even fewer things can open your eyes to just how helpless you are when sickness invades the life you once took for granted." Arlene remembered the nodding heads of the group. Their reserved, exhausted faces.

She had decided that she would not be returning to work, knowing she needed to be available for her family. The advice she always preached began rattling through her mind with relentless intensity. Take care of yourself. Lean on others for help. Accept your limitations. But these notions were overpowered by a surge of what-ifs. What if we couldn't receive the necessary support during the pandemic? What if the cancer was spreading too rapidly to stop — or even slow down? What if Harvey needed to be hospitalized? What if we were in this alone?

The questions bubbled. And with these boiling concerns came a realization that was difficult to accept: she was no longer just the facilitator of a support group. At fifty-nine, she was now a caregiver herself.

After a wave of anxiety passed — it always came in waves — she turned off the TV and inhaled deeply, remembering what she'd always told her groups, a repeated analogy about airplane passengers in an emergency, one that was as clichéd as it was valid. "Before you can help a fellow passenger, you need to put on your own oxygen mask."

Of course, Arlene knew that caring for yourself when you want to save someone else is easier said than done. The responsibility-induced anxieties a caregiver can accumulate are often intensified by sleepless nights, struggles to organize medication, and general emotional fatigue. The heroic narratives in books or movies don't shine much light on the self-care needed to sustain such arduous efforts, preferring instead to spotlight the selfless lover who falls asleep on a chair next to a hospital bed, the exhausted husband or wife who hasn't eaten in days and buzzes with caffeine and boundless devotion, ready to suffocate themselves if it means giving their ill spouse another breath of air. Arlene wasn't going to let herself suffocate. She inhaled a deep breath.

She adored Harvey, and she told herself that she would do whatever it took to make him better. He was her best friend. Her soulmate, whatever that meant. But she knew that to be the best help possible, she needed to make a plan. A plan that utilized the many healthcare workers in the family. A plan that would make this gruelling situation easier. She would be the captain of the ship, guiding us into an unforgiving storm, a storm she'd spent a career navigating from afar.

The thought of her own father's death flashed briefly through her mind, but she pushed the memory away and tried to stay centred. She knew what she'd do.

She'd let the moments pour in, one after the other, embracing the time she had left with the man she loved and had built a life with.

Responding to each catastrophe in isolation, she'd find solace in the little victories. The relief and joy. The sunny mornings and peaceful evenings. The moments where life stands still. By doing this, she'd turn the totality of what awaited, the drowning waves of despair, into smaller ripples of turmoil.

Benjamin Button
April 2020

"Anything else?"

"Not really."

"So, it was just a normal, small-town childhood?"

"Pretty much."

"Can you tell me more about your parents?"

"What do you want to know?"

"Anything …"

"You know … I was fourteen when my mom died and it was … really sad. Twenty-two when my dad died and it was … well … also sad."

"What was your mother like?"

"She was nice."

That's when the expected happened. With the mere mention of his mother, Dad turned away on the bed, facing the window and the afternoon sunlight filtering through blinds. The grandmother I never knew was a topic of discussion he routinely avoided, and today was no exception. Sometimes, I figured, a whirlwind of emotions and memories are condensed to single, simplistic adjectives.

I hit pause on my iPhone that rested on the nightstand. The problem wasn't solely how guarded Dad was or the vagueness of his responses, but more that I wasn't sure what questions to ask. I wanted to reach him, but I wasn't sure how. What could I possibly ask now that I'd want to ask him in the future — when I couldn't?

In journalism school, we unpacked the art of the interview — the subtle and nuanced techniques for probing for details and getting someone talking. The sympathetic nods, the fluff comments to break the ice, the softball questions to build rapport, mirrored body language, affirmative statements, and so on. But any skills I had acquired over the years became irrelevant as I sat in the spare bedroom on the carpet next to Dad's bed. In the interview that mattered most, I was choking. It didn't help that I was questioning my toughest source yet.

After ten minutes of surface-level responses to inquiries about his childhood, Dad turned on Netflix. "We'll continue this later," he said.

We'd been ploughing through an endless stream of movies together. Recently we watched *The Curious Case of Benjamin Button*. The part at the end when Brad Pitt's character decides to leave his family seemed to bother him deeply.

"I just don't get it," Dad said.

"What?"

"Why would he leave?"

"He doesn't want to be a burden for his wife and daughter," I said. "His age is rapidly reversing, and he doesn't want to be a helpless baby that they have to take care of. He wants to keep the memory of himself intact."

"No … he's leaving his daughter before she's three years old, before she could even remember him. He's leaving before any lasting memories can form."

"Maybe it's easier that way," I said.

"It doesn't make any sense," he said, scratching his head. "If he really loved them, he'd stay as long as he could."

I wondered if there was something revealing about his past hidden in this reaction. I had heard that Dad stayed home with his mother the summer she died, when his two siblings were off at a sleep-away camp, travelling back home every weekend. I didn't know the details of her decline. But I did know — though not yet from first-hand experience — that terminal illness has a way of reversing the age of the patient, rendering them, eventually, as helpless and dependent as an infant. Maybe, though, seeing her that way was preferable to not having her in his life at all.

Over the years, I had grown accustomed to being forced to guess what Dad was feeling. He had always been a devoted father, ready to drop everything for his family, prepared to drive any distance, wait out any line, spend any dollar to enrich or benefit our lives, but, often, he could seem distracted. Whenever he was stressed, his jaw would tense, and he'd scratch his scalp and pace around whatever room was dominated by legal files.

His work, after all, was another way for him to show his devotion to us; it offered the means for providing us with financial security and the small luxuries of a middle-class life. But he normally seemed unwilling to share with us whatever was going on in his head, preferring to keep his anxieties locked up. In place of emotional vulnerability, he'd unload a long-winded rant about a recent case, a convoluted monologue filled with legal jargon that was impossible for my younger self to decipher. When I was growing up, this sometimes made conversations with him difficult.

But movies have long been our space of togetherness. With movies, nothing needs to be said. Nothing should be said as you escape into the story flashing across the screen. With a box of popcorn and squeaky theatre seats, being next to him was the only necessity. When I was twelve, he took me to see *Casino Royale*, the first James Bond film with Daniel Craig. It was a franchise Dad was always fond of, especially the Sean Connery originals, and we spent twenty minutes after the credits running around the Cineplex parking lot, ducking behind parked cars with finger guns, pretending to be double-0 agents on a mission.

When he'd pose and point that finger gun, he'd say the iconic line: "Bond. James Bond." (His British accent always sounded Indian.) Often, our best moments were when we both became a couple of kids running around. During these sprees of play, Dad's age would reverse, like Benjamin Button's.

When accelerating on the highway, he'd sometimes turn to me and say, "All right, Mitch, time for your *Fast and Furious* audition. I'm gonna need you to open your door and jump onto that passing truck. Then you're gonna have to smash open the windshield, decapitate the driver, and get off at the next exit. Easy, right? Okay, on three. One, two, three!"

As the reality of his illness began to manifest itself, I was afraid that the sporadic playfulness that was so common in his personality was beginning to fade. The palliative team had prescribed twenty-milligram morphine tabs for the excruciating pain in his rectum, and they normally knocked him out before we could finish each movie. Drowsiness had joined agony as a constant companion in Dad's post-diagnosis life.

As he drifted off to sleep, I closed the door softly, squeezing my iPhone tightly, wondering how many more chances I'd get to ask the deeper questions, and how many more movies would fill the silence of answers unsaid.

Information
April 2020

Days after Uncle Earl learned about his brother's diagnosis, he sat in his home office and dove into the medical literature.

A neurologist who practises in downtown Toronto, Earl has travelled all over the world to attend international research conferences, and his home office is decorated with knick-knacks brought back from his extensive excursions. (A particular mask he got from Bali, mounted on the wall before a pull-out couch — where I once slept after a night of binge-watching *The Lord of the Rings* trilogy — gave my ten-year-old self nightmares.)

"I have the hair; Earl has the height," Dad would always say. He was closer to five foot eight; Uncle Earl hit about six foot three (and had a little less hair). Well-dressed, often wearing thick-rimmed glasses that complete his intelligent demeanour, Earl is a man of composure and logic. He recognizes the value of information. And, as he felt heartsick for his younger brother, information is what he reached for.

"Anorectal malignant melanoma (AMM) is a rare and aggressive malignancy with poor prognosis, yet no consensus of treatment exists to date," read one case report in a medical journal published within the last decade. "In general, the five-year survival rate is low, being only 6 percent to 22 percent reportedly with a median survival period of 12.2 to 22 months."

Another medical article, which detailed a study of British patients with all stages of the disease, listed a five-year survival rate of only 14 percent. It also reported a median survival duration of less than ten months after being diagnosed. Treatments, according to the literature, were currently confined to immunotherapy, targeted radiation, and surgical removal of tumours — all of these became increasingly more complicated during late-stage metastasization. Advancements in clinical studies promised new therapeutic frontiers for patients diagnosed with the more typical cutaneous melanoma, the most common type of melanoma cancer, often caused by overexposure to the sun, but treatments for the rare subgroup of patients with mucosal melanoma, the kind Harvey had, which has no known cause, remained undeveloped and unexplored.

In these findings, Earl's rational mind saw limited hope. *Maybe Harv has another year left*, my uncle thought to himself. *Maybe a couple years. Maybe more promising treatments will arrive, giving him a little more time.*

But the truth was painfully apparent in the file of medical articles Earl printed off: this disease would probably kill his brother.

This was something Harvey didn't appear to fully recognize. He had seemed hopeful on the phone, claiming to be "lucky" that the problem was identified before it was too late. Earl was beginning to see just how unlucky his younger brother was.

Shouldering this knowledge, he knew there wasn't much he could do, except what always came naturally: be there for his family. Show up in whatever way they need him. Provide whatever support he could. But he was another healthcare professional amid a global pandemic, and the necessity of physical distance would stand in the way of him acting on his brotherly instincts.

On a shelf in Uncle Earl's TV room, outside his home office, is a vast collection of family photos — pictures of his four nephews, his only niece, his brother-in-law, sister-in-law, and his two siblings. Smiling faces from younger days, joyful moments, happier times.

There are also photos of his parents — Max, with handsome features and a warm smile, and Sandra, with brown eyes and curly hair. These were the grandparents I never knew.

After losing them at a young age, he and his two siblings stuck together. They started a new life, built on the foundation of love their parents had left behind. Togetherness had gotten them through dark times. It did then. But could it now, when distance was required?

As he closed the file of medical research, Uncle Earl could only hope so.

Fallout Shelter
April 2020

Aunt Louise poured the kettle's hot water, and steam bloomed out of the teacup. On the counter next to it lay a copy of the *Toronto Star* newspaper from March 17. A column headed "Doctors and nurses are on the front lines …" mentioned her husband, Howard, and their son Daniel. A father and son deep in the trenches of the city's medical battle.

The piece, written by columnist Bruce Arthur, had a Hemingway-esque simplicity to it — full of commas and short sentences, with a few choice quotes sprinkled throughout:

He's proud of his son. His son tells him, you can't go to work, you're 72, you work three shifts in the ER, you can't go. You're the high-risk population, I'll pay your salary. Howard is currently in self-isolation after cutting short a Florida vacation.

"I have a shift scheduled at the hospital," Howard says. "I still do emergency. I may go do it. I don't think the family will approve, but it's what I've been doing for 40 years."

In 2003 he had direct contact with a SARS patient who died. He isn't nervous about this yet, he says. Like everyone else, he thinks the storm is coming.

"Daniel graduated from high school, and I was on the lawn across the road from the party," Howard says. "Because I wasn't allowed off my property. But at that time, they told me I could go to work as long as I wore a mask. We didn't know as much then.... You sound young. You ever see *Hill Street Blues*? Let's be careful out there."

This is life before wartime. There are a lot of people who are going to fight.

It was published weeks before Dad's diagnosis. Despite his printed quotes, Uncle Howie would ultimately choose not to report to ER; new family priorities would shift his focus.

❖

Louise was a wife and mother — and social worker — who was already worried about her husband and son before her brother got terminal cancer. She wished she could protect her whole family, keep them together and safe. She felt overwhelmed by the unpredictability of everything. The feeling reminded her of when she was twelve and obsessed with fallout shelters.

She knew it wasn't typical, her young fixation with such extreme safety — but how else would her family be protected from the threat of a nuclear attack by the Soviet Union? She recalled the Cold War paranoia that plagued the world all those years ago, the widespread fear that, at any time, a tidal wave of radioactive ash could bury everything she knew and loved.

When she was young, twelve or thirteen, maybe, she once forged her mother's signature on the request slip for a fallout shelter construction plan, which she had ripped out of a recent issue of *Good Housekeeping*. The advertisement for the family-sized nuclear fallout shelter, with thirty-centimetre-thick concrete walls, a filtered air system, and a rolled-steel door with thick rubber gasket, was a perfect solution to her anxieties. In the ad, the slogan *Protect your family!* was printed beneath a cartoon image of an atomic mushroom explosion.

Now, more than fifty years later, Louise found herself longing for protection, for cover, yet again. She knew the concrete walls of a fallout shelter wouldn't stop the deadly virus or the cancer growing in her brother. But she desperately wanted to keep her family together and close. She was willing to do whatever it took to make it possible.

"There are a lot of people who are going to fight," read the last line of that column. But there was a fight within the fight now, and she was afraid what might happen if her brother got left behind.

Chair Screech
April 2020

Daniel began the intubation process in the negative-pressure operating room. It was a complicated and invasive procedure, involving the administration of paralytic drugs and the insertion of a tube down an eighty-year-old woman's airway.

Next to him were two nurses — one to record the process and one to gather medicine and equipment. Another nurse stood at the door outside. There was also a respiratory therapist, in charge of mitigating the risk that came with the patient's every breath.

He kept his eyes on the screen. It showed a video transmission from the laryngoscope he was tightly holding, a metal tool equipped with a small camera to help guide the airway tube between the vocal cords. The patient's oxygen levels were shown on an adjacent monitor. Daniel knew that each movement had to be measured, deliberate — a single cough would send virus particles flying over his face shield.

Many Toronto hospitals had deployed intubation teams that specialized in aerosol management, but Mississauga

Hospital, the facility west of Toronto where Daniel worked, had chosen to allow some of their more confident emergency physicians to hold the laryngoscope. Daniel was capable of meeting the challenge.

He had intubated patients many times before, but, today, he was a little distracted. Daniel tried to push the thought of his uncle out of his mind and focus on the elderly woman lying beneath him. The infected patient was the third nursing home senior he had intubated that month — the emergency room had seen a flood of Covid-19 patients from long-term care homes. In other parts of the country, he had heard, such patients were pushing hospitals to overcapacity.

A few days prior, Daniel had treated two elderly patients who came into the emergency room without end-of-life instructions. He spent over an hour tracking down their families and getting them on the phone. If the hospital was busier, he knew that they likely would've been left totally out of the loop, and the decisions about resuscitation and compressions would've been up to him. In all the chaos of the health crisis, Daniel knew that the only thing worse than dying without your family was dying without your family knowing about it. And the latter had become a common occurrence during his emergency shifts. The absence of loved ones during a patient's final moments left an emptiness in the room that was impossible to fill. The physicians charged with caring for these patients were forced to shoulder a crippling burden of responsibility.

Daniel carefully threaded the tube down the woman's windpipe, avoiding her esophagus, connecting it to her lungs. The ventilator hummed mechanically. Daniel listened to the rhythm of inhalation and exhalation, the flow of aided breath.

"Good job, everyone," he said shortly after the job was done. He removed his latex gloves and squirted some hand sanitizer out of a wall dispenser. Then he walked down the hall and stepped into the staff lounge for a moment — to check his phone and take a breath.

There were a few messages from Aunt Arlene, and he responded immediately. They were simple questions about morphine spacing and whether Lyrica could be taken with meals. He had been trying not to dwell on his uncle's illness, but with every patient he saw, Uncle Harvey's face came to mind.

Daniel remembered the last time he saw Harvey in person, at the time of his own dad's seventy-second birthday celebration, at that Italian restaurant midtown. The moment Daniel arrived, some of the family screeched their chairs a little farther away. "Very funny," he said, as he and his girlfriend (and future wife), Jenna, joined the long wooden table near the back of the brightly lit pizzeria. It was a cold Friday night in early March, weeks before the world shut down.

The chair-screech greeting was a response to what Daniel had learned a couple days prior. The clinical lead of the hospital's emergency department had called, informing him that two of his recent patients were among Canada's first to test positive for Covid-19. His father, Uncle Howie, had phoned to warn everyone hours before his birthday celebration. He explained that while Daniel had worn all the PPE required, he had offered to sit this one out if we didn't feel comfortable. Nobody was really concerned. As far as we knew, this virus was nothing out of the ordinary. And togetherness was something this family was slow to let go of.

Ambient conversations — likely about hand sanitizer or toilet paper — filled the restaurant. Laughter, applause, a baby wailing, glasses clinking, cutlery scraping plates — all of it articulating a space buzzing with people, noise that only weeks later would seem like the mark of a different time. Daniel's brother, Sandon, did his Bernie Sanders impersonation. Uncle Earl talked about a recent trip to Italy. Harvey told a joke but butchered the punchline. Louise FaceTimed her grandson in Ottawa. Howie blew out the candles. Steph talked about how Ryan couldn't make it again, how exhausted he was from residency — the demands of which were intimately understood at the table.

Everyone sat less than a foot apart. Looking back, Daniel, like everyone, wished he had appreciated that closeness a little more. Enduring the storm of medical decisions and the emotional toll that comes with helping patients in critical condition, he has always counted on family to keep him centred.

After putting his phone away, he adjusted his fresh mask, sucked in some air, and walked back onto the emergency room floor.

Pain in the Ass
April 20, 2020

"I made a living as a personal injury lawyer, as a pain in people's ass — now I'm making a living from having a pain in the ass," Dad said to every person who called him to express their concern.

The hit-or-miss joke referred to the long-term disability insurance he filed for — monthly compensation that made it possible for him to happily retire and live comfortably without continuing his law firm. The money would keep coming until he turned seventy. He just needed to live that long. And that part, we were about to learn, wasn't so simple.

Dr. Teresa Petrella, wearing a mask and face shield, entered the bright room in Sunnybrook Hospital. She was a tall woman in her fifties, with friendly blue eyes and brown hair. "How are you feeling today, Harvey?"

"Not bad," he said.

Courtesy of Covid restrictions, Dad had to endure his first oncology meeting alone, without any family by his side. As he sat on a reclinable chair, he tried to look calm. In his hands, he carried a binder of family photos Mom had assembled, including one of our eighty-three-pound goldendoodle, Charley. (Around three in the morning he had printed the photos off from his iPad.)

"I heard you have some family that wanted to call in for this," Dr. Petrella said shortly after her greeting. "You can go ahead and patch them in now."

Hoping to take notes and help hack through the medical jargon that riddles the path through treatment, the doctors of our family attempted to join the call. What followed was a cascade of technical difficulties, successfully breaking the tension of the moment.

"Hi ... can you hear me?"

"Hello? Hello?"

"Howie ... you can't hear? Try increasing the volume ..."

Dr. Petrella was accustomed to having one or two family members call in during these Covid-restricted meetings. She was less accustomed to having the intimate and emotionally draining briefings turn into an eight-person conference call. As she would later tell me, the fact that the majority of these family members were also medical professionals made it all the more unusual.

"Hi, Dr. Petrella, this is Harvey's nephew, Daniel ... I'm an emergency physician at Mississauga Hospital."

"Howard, here ... Harvey's brother-in-law ...: I'm an emergency physician at Scarborough General."

"Hi, Arlene again ... Harvey's wife ... I'm not a doctor; I'm a social worker. I'd also like my daughter, a registered dietitian, and her boyfriend to join the call ... he's a general surgery resident ... one minute ..."

"Lots of healthcare workers in the family," Dr. Petrella mused out loud.

Dad nodded. "We also have a journalist." (He never failed to bring that up.)

Eventually, after the wave of introductions, Dr. Petrella launched into the details, including much of what we already suspected.

Advanced stage mucosal melanoma had spread to my father's liver, lymph nodes, and lungs. He was eligible for immunotherapy. Chemo wouldn't help, especially given the liver metastasization. Targeted radiation could shrink the primary tumour on his rectum, and might control the bleeding, but surgery would delay the overall treatment plan. Alternative pain management solutions would be considered with the palliative team. (*Palliative* was a scary word.) Biomarkers, which were lab tests intended to determine whether or not the melanoma mutation would respond to certain drug therapies, were in process. Bone scans were required, as was more blood work. A lot was unknown. But what *was* known was this: it didn't look good.

We were dealing with advanced stage melanoma cancer that started in his rectum and had reached Stage 4 metastasization. Less than 1 percent of melanoma cancers are anorectal, so not only was this extremely rare, it was, given the lack of therapeutic trials, unusually complicated. And cancer is *always* complicated.

Daniel asked questions about clinical trials of drugs that could stand as potential contingency options. Dr. Petrella explained that it was too early to tell if any were a possibility with Dad's current condition and maintained that immunotherapy was our best option. The physicians of my family knew there was little evidence that suggested any treatment would work for this type of malignancy.

"Well, all we can do is our best," Dad said, and a long silence filled the line. Distant sniffles were just audible beneath the crackle and hum of phone speakers. There are some moments of silence that last only a few seconds but feel like an hour. This was one of those moments.

At the end of the meeting, after everyone hung up, Dad told Dr. Petrella his hit-or-miss joke. "You know, I made a living as a personal injury lawyer, as a pain in people's ass. Now I'm making a living by *having* a pain in the ass!"

He couldn't tell if she smiled behind her face mask.

Elias
April 2020

Sunlight rippled through the windshield, and with the driver's seat cranked back and my feet propped up on the steering wheel, I sat with my thumbs tapping my iPhone screen.

I was waiting in the east parking lot of the Sunnybrook Melanoma Clinic, finishing that feature story for the *Walrus* about families of healthcare workers. After accessing my interview transcriptions online, I was writing a rough draft on my phone's Google Docs app, finding solace in letting the words spill out of me without self-scrutiny, without that inner critic that often stops writers from writing. Dumping the words on my phone seemed to dissolve the pressure that always came with typing on my laptop. I had forgotten how good it felt to just let it all flow out.

I remembered, briefly, that feeling of inadequacy I experienced shortly after the editor from the *Walrus* approved the pitch I emailed, weeks before I discovered Dad's illness. I was paralyzed by the eagerness to do a good job; filling a blank page became my sole focus, and I put in hours of effort trying to create a perfect piece. Looking back, I realized how excessive my second-guessing of myself was, how much time I spent in my own head. And then suddenly, a larger tragedy had snapped me out of my daze and made all previous struggles seem so manageable.

Despite my father's cancer dominating my mind, I still recognized an urge, an obligation, maybe, to do right by my sources — the people I had interviewed. One Toronto emergency physician I spoke to was living in an Airbnb apartment separate from his family, only seeing them for occasional weekend walks during which they would keep the necessary distance. His wife, who I also interviewed, said their youngest son often burst into tears after their father said goodbye on those walks, the uncertainty of not knowing the next time he'd see his dad taking its toll. I knew such sacrifices and isolation from their families were all too common for healthcare workers during this historic moment, and I wanted to play my role in articulating that common experience.

Also, sitting in that parking lot for more than three hours, I knew there wasn't much else to do but take emotional refuge in the distraction of my work. There was doing that, or letting my mind spiral, which I opted to avoid. I chose to be productive, to tackle my peripheral tasks first, so I could later focus, exclusively, on the main challenge.

Eventually, Dad knocked on the window, and I unlocked the car and threw my phone aside. Still wearing his mask, he climbed in and closed the door, looking forward. Seatbelts clicked. I readjusted my seat, turned on the ignition, and began the drive home.

Daniel had sent the family an email summarizing the details of the meeting, so I already knew what was on Dad's mind: the side effects of immunotherapy, the statistical likelihood of the treatment working, the targeted radiation that could slow the spread of the primary tumour and might alleviate the pain, the metastasized cancer throughout his liver and lungs. The unlikely, possibly non-existent, chance of survival.

With tree branches budding leaves on Bayview Avenue, it felt like we were driving through a sick juxtaposition: the start of spring, and the end of Dad's life. It was one of those moments when you want time to stop.

Trying to distract both of us, I played our favourite road trip song: "Elias," by Dispatch. The music poured from the stereo as we accelerated down the road.

"Elias" was first released in 1996. It's about a man from Zimbabwe, named Elias, who Dispatch guitarist and singer Chad Urmston — also known as Chadwick Stokes — met while visiting the country in 1994. Elias and his family lived in Section 17, one of Zimbabwe's most heavily HIV/AIDS infected regions. At the time of the song's release, about 8,500 new people were being infected each day in Zimbabwe and over 6,000 deaths from the disease were being recorded daily.

The first three verses are chanted in Shona, a language spoken in Zimbabwe. The first verse speaks of friendship and how, when you're feeling an absence of hope, you shouldn't be afraid to lean on your friends to lift you up. The second verse includes a customary greeting in Zimbabwe. "*Makasimba*" translates to "Are you strong?" The response to this is: "I am strong if you are strong." And then the greeter replies confidently, "I am strong."

As he sat in the passenger's seat, Dad's foot started tapping to the music. Then, as the guitar chords joined the harmony and the beat picked up, his hand started patting his knee and his head started bobbing. A smile found my face because I knew what was coming. As he started drumming the glove compartment, I bumped the volume for the English chorus, and Dad belted the words with all his tone-deaf enthusiasm:

> Hold my hand just one more time
> To see if you're really going to meet me
> Hold my hand just one more time
> To see if you're really gonna meet me

I sang the next verse with him (equally off-key). Keeping one hand on the steering wheel, I extended my arm to the passenger seat. Dad took my hand and squeezed it tight.

Branches swayed a little slower as we sang the rest of that song together. And as we belted the lyrics, the weight of our circumstances seemed to dissolve. Each breath felt a little more satisfying. Each sound, a little more beautiful.

With unexpected joy, we drove down the open road, uncertain of what awaited, thankful for car rides and loud music and the time we still had.

A Sanctuary of Imagination
June 1963

"Bond," Sean Connery said, sitting behind a casino table crowded with stacks of chips, tobacco smoke coiling around him. "James Bond."

The large auditorium was alive with people slurping drinks and chewing popcorn. Sitting next to his siblings, with his father running the front door and his mother working the snack bar in the lobby behind, Harvey was comforted by the familiarity of all of it — the clicking of the projector's gears, the ray of light streaming through darkness onto the screen, the dust particles hovering in the glow.

To some, the family-owned movie theatre was a sacred environment, a place of community where the people of the small town sat back to forget their lives for a couple hours and escape into an exotic world. To look through the eyes of someone else — someone bigger, bolder, more adventurous. The town movie theatre was more than a place that offered entertainment: it was a sanctuary for the imagination. As you sat there, you could be anyone.

The theatre opened a decade before the new blockbuster release about a spy with a licence to kill. It was an ordinary day in 1948, when a pair of newlyweds were driving from Ottawa, down Highway 17, on their way to Timmins. Needing to take a break, they stopped at a small town buzzing with activity.

There was a hydroelectric dam being built in the area — it would become the Otto Holden Generating Station — and it was bringing in hordes of construction workers and their families. It seemed like a promising location for business. Max and Sandra, the grandparents I never knew, decided that Mattawa, Ontario, needed a sanctuary for the townspeople's imaginations.

Max's family had been building and operating movie theatres in a number of towns in northern Ontario for the previous decade, catering films to Canadians otherwise starved of cinematic access. It was a formula Max and Sandra intended to replicate. With the plan of utilizing construction material from Sandra's family, who ran a lumber company in Timmins, they purchased the property and broke ground.

The plan was to stay for only a year, just to get the place up and running. But months before the theatre was complete, Louise was born, and the couple that became a family stayed where they were. A year later, Earl joined the family, and a year after that came Harvey.

For the first couple of months of Harvey's life, he and his family lived in an apartment on top of the movie theatre. It was cozy and well-furnished. They lived in that apartment until their parents decided to settle the clan more permanently a few streets over in a modern home, which they designed and built, with big windows, a dishwasher, and a large backyard with a vegetable garden.

On nights of new releases, the family would head to the theatre together, walking through the backyard gateway and across the street, Quebec's Laurentian Mountains looming over them, the Mattawa River glimmering moonlight at the edge of town.

I try my best to picture it: the only Jewish family in a small community — three siblings no more than three years apart. A mother with big brown eyes and curly hair. A father with handsome features and a warm smile. I wish I knew more than that. The truth is, though, my grandparents remain a mystery. All I've been able to gather are the fragmented details my aunt, uncle, and father had been willing to provide.

Sandra had a degree from Queen's University and was one of the administrators of the local library. She always emphasized education and challenged her kids to strive for their best, to think critically about the world around them. The relationship between my dad and Sandra was special, my aunt and uncle would tell me, in a way that a mother's relationship with her youngest often is.

Max was president of the town's Lion Club and chair of the school board. He travelled frequently to Toronto to negotiate booking releases. Soft-spoken, gentle, and well-dressed, he conveyed a natural elegance. Louise would tell me she has a foggy recollection of her father once playing records by Jewish musicians, collections of songs composed during the

Holocaust, as if to show that beautiful things can emerge out of dark times.

But the larger details of what Max and Sandra stood for, how they loved their children, who they really were, have remained inaccessible to me — all I have is my imagination. Only with it can I visualize the two people my dad lost too young. A specific scene comes to mind.

I imagine my dad sitting in the theatre, next to his mother, feeling the security that comes with being in a familiar place. It's years before they would move to Toronto, before the doctors would discover the tumours on Sandra's liver, before they'd investigate the lumps on Max's neck.

James Bond is throwing punches. That projector is clicking above. I see her glimpse at her younger son in the auditorium's glow. I like to believe that when she looked at him Harvey felt like he could achieve greatness. That he could become anyone he chose to be.

I see a young smile curving on his face. He's enthralled by Sean Connery's performance — his snappy dialogue, brute force, adventurous spirit. He's happy. He's safe. He's in a place of love, caught in a rare flicker between the past and future, untouched by the torments of grief and loss.

I see Sandra grab her son's hand beneath a basket of popcorn, gripping the moment before it passes away.

Part Two:
The Universal Language

Old Life
April 2020

Boxes were stacked on top of one another, dust billowed, and *The Lion King*'s "I Just Can't Wait to Be King" reverberated through my downtown apartment.

I had abandoned it in early March, believing, like everyone else, that the pandemic would be over in a few weeks and I'd return before the end of my final semester of my master's in journalism degree. Those were the days when my biggest problem was submitting story drafts on time to the editors at the student magazine I worked for or completing a final assignment before the deadline.

I had already been living there for more than a year, so I was able to terminate the lease with two months' notice. Shortly after learning about my dad's diagnosis, my two buddies Coby and Tal, wearing masks and keeping their distance, helped me stack plastic boxes and clear out cabinets and closets.

Coby was playing the music and had been abruptly switching from rap, to rock, to the *Lion King* soundtrack. He clapped his hands loudly to the beat as Simba sang about the freedoms of kingship and Tal emptied the fridge.

"You taking these?" Tal asked, pointing to a few beers left on the door shelf.

"I'm pretty sure they've been there since September," I admitted.

"Apple cider, anyone?"

After dragging my mattress out of my room, I collapsed onto the couch, next to a duffle bag of clothes, and gazed out the window. Tears blurred my vision.

"You okay?" Coby asked me, lowering the volume on his phone.

"I just can't believe how much has changed in a month," I said, still looking out the window. "Not just with my dad ... With everything."

"I know," Coby said. "It's all just ... unbelievable."

Coby was there the night we learned Gaby died. He was one of the fraternity brothers offering comfort and crying into shoulders at the frat house. The two of us were supposed to move in together at the end of the summer, but now it was obvious that wasn't going to happen. It was another reminder how suddenly plans, just like life, can end.

Once the apartment was finally cleared out, I walked around the empty space, feeling a longing for that time in my life when everything was normal. A longing for independence and freedom, for those mornings where I'd look out at the cityscape and believe that life could only get better and that limitless possibilities awaited. I'd conquer this town with my words, I decided long ago, indulging in the delusions of ego. Write my way to the top of this concrete jungle. Work hard and use sentences to build a life — paragraphs would be my building blocks. I'd write books. Dad would show up at signings. He'd pat me on the back with that big smile and say, "Knew it! Always knew it!" It felt like a promise fading before my eyes.

Before I moved in there, I was away for my undergraduate degree in a different city. I hadn't lived full-time in my parent's house for more than seven years, and, admittedly, I felt like my return would be like travelling backward on a path I had already walked. But I knew that there was nowhere else I was supposed to be. I knew there weren't many moments in life when such belonging could anchor me.

We spend so much of our early twenties stumbling toward forks in the path, going left when we should've gone right, contemplating decision after decision, life choice after life choice. Directions have never been my forte. So, I guess it was relieving to find myself on a one-way street, a single, bumpy road that would lead me nowhere but home.

After leaving the key on the counter, I walked out of the empty apartment and closed the door on my old life.

Photos on the Wall
April 2020

The ulcerated tumour was identified to be on the most sensitive part of Dad's rectum. Whenever he needed to pass a stool, he risked filling the toilet bowl with blood.

Since his diagnosis, he had been trying different medications to stop the problem, but they hadn't helped the pain. Morphine made him spacey and constipated — this ended up hurting him more — but it was also the only remedy that made the constant agony bearable. Despite this, he never complained.

Mom had started making charts to document Dad's pain levels — ten being the highest, one the lowest. Even with the morphine, he was never under four. As he lay on his bed, enduring all this torment, Dad worried about one of his clients who had suffered severe head trauma in a car accident. He stressed over the case, saying that he wanted to settle it while he still could. Even gravely ill, he was consumed by the desire to help someone in need.

Whenever he got a call from a friend, he forced a smile and pretended he was perfectly okay. "Not bad, not bad" was his automatic response when someone asked him how he was doing. He had been telling his "pain in the ass" joke over and over again, desperate to make light of something so heavy, to bring comfort to others. But I knew that, deep down, he felt the joke had stopped being funny a while ago.

The healthcare professionals in the family made suggestions, all of which were reviewed and many of which were approved by Dad's "most responsible physicians" (known as MRPs), Dr. Petrella and the palliative care team. Uncle Howie had suggested Zofran for nausea, a condition that is inevitably experienced by those with elevated levels of liver enzymes. Steph had sent us nutritional supplement drinks to compensate for Dad's weight loss. Daniel had recommended increasing the midday morphine dose by fifteen milligrams and suggested Lyrica for nerve pain. He was looking into THC (cannabis-based) alternatives. Uncle Norman had begun calling in regularly to check Dad's vitals and began helping Daniel research pain management options. Despite us being physically apart, our team was coming together. "Avengers Assemble!" Dad would call between morphine-induced micro-naps.

While the chaotic collaboration of family members strove to keep him comfortable, Mom made extra efforts to keep Dad's spirits up, to maintain his typical optimism. She started printing off photos of family members and taping them to the walls of the spare bedroom where he was sleeping.

One picture had the four of us out for dinner somewhere, wearing winter jackets in a dimly lit restaurant lobby. Another showed Steph and me as little kids at one of her dance recitals, me with the rambunctious smirk of a child up to no good, her with a face caked in show makeup. There was one with Steph and Dad standing on a summer evening, the orange glow of a setting sun illuminating their smiles as Steph rested her head on her father's shoulder.

"She'll be home soon," I told Dad, as I noticed his glassy eyes settling on that picture.

"I know," he said, adjusting his head on a pillow. "I can't wait."

✦

Steph hesitated before walking in the front door, carrying a box of nutritional supplement drinks under one arm.

Over the previous days, she did what she could to prevent being exposed to the virus and tried, as much as was possible, to distance herself from Ryan in their shared condo. But there were limits to how completely she could isolate herself, and, therefore, there were risks to her entry.

Steph decided that she would keep her distance from the family despite living in the house, at least for the first week. Wearing a mask that covered most of her small face, she'd eat her meals at a different table, use the downstairs bathroom, and avoid giving anyone a hug for the time being.

This distance would apply to all but one family member. As she walked in, Charley gave Steph the devoted greeting every good dog feels obliged to give. His tail wagged like a high-speed windshield wiper, and his long body wobbled and vibrated, as if he was having an ecstatic experience in the presence of the Messiah. As Steph scratched his head, he leaned against her, burying his muzzle into her leg, elated and thankful for her return.

"Dad's sleeping upstairs," Mom called, blowing her daughter a kiss from the kitchen with a phone shouldered against her ear, two pill containers clenched in one hand. "Welcome home!"

Dads Who Dance in Underwear Society
April 2020

There is an ancient brotherhood of fathers who sporadically dance in their underwear around their house. My dad was a secret member.

It never mattered the song, because those sporadic convulsions of movement excused as dancing didn't follow much rhythm, anyway. Or, one could say, they followed a rhythm exclusive to the Dads Who Dance in Underwear Society.

This is a secret society that exists in households worldwide. Membership isn't exclusive. It includes any dad with the vigour, zest, and ill-advised confidence to shake their ass while attired in minimum clothing, to jubilantly swing hips and strum air guitars, to rock to the tunes of Van Morrison, The Beatles, Elvis Presley, or any musician who inspires the mood.

Accessories for these performative rituals were, in my father's case, limited. All that was needed was a pair of tighty-whities or baggy boxers — any conceivable underwear would do. Sometimes a makeshift hat was balanced on his head — a roll of toilet paper, a pillow, a spatula, anything that could further rouse audience laughter. Because the number one objective of the Dads Who Dance in Underwear Society is exactly that: make your audience laugh. And, in fulfilling that objective, my dad was a never-failing hit.

Most people didn't know this side of Dad. Outside of the house, he was often serious and stoic, quick with a joke, yes, but definitely not someone to bust out freestyle dance moves without clothes. He was a calculated and logic-oriented personal injury lawyer beyond our front door, but inside our family walls, he was an underwear-flaunting rockstar.

Energized by Steph's return, Dad danced around the upstairs hallway in his boxers. With arms swinging, head bobbing, and legs bouncing, he moved to the music booming from the spare bedroom. His dance numbers diffused all tension in the house, got my mom, sister, and me roaring on the floor, convulsed by deep belly giggles that made us choke and gasp.

Our response, as always, only further provoked him; he lunged and raised an arm like a ballerina, then crouched low like a ski racer rocketing down a slope. He pointed a fist like Freddie Mercury. And when he played Shakira's "Hips Don't Lie," we lost it even more.

Here was a man in the throes of terminal cancer thrusting his hips to Shakira with the fiery passion of a Latin ballroom dancer, wearing a pair of baggy boxers instead of a ruby suit, fuelled by the tear-inducing laughter of his applauding wife and kids.

Life doesn't get stranger than this.

❋

Upon returning to an empty condo after a long hospital shift, Ryan called Stephanie on FaceTime. When she answered, he thought at first she was crying but soon realized she was laughing so hard she had tears. Her dad was dancing around the house again.

When Steph giggled, her blue eyes smiled and her nose wrinkled. Her laugh was infectious.

"Miss you," Ryan said, his twelve-hour-shift exhaustion apparent on the grainy screen.

"Miss you, too," she replied.

Mailman
April 2020

After the targeted radiation, Dad suffered frequent bowel urgency, which made it difficult for him to sleep through the night. Every hour, he jolted out of bed and sprinted to the washroom. He had started using adult diapers.

I lay awake at night, waiting to hear the groan of the floorboard outside of his room, ready to snap up and help him. His liver enzymes had been steadily increasing, and he was becoming more nauseated and disoriented. I was worried he'd fall. Mom was, too, and she left a note on the hallway wall before the staircase: *Don't go downstairs without help! Love you!*

(Mom was the notorious note writer in our family. When we were growing up, she'd cover our walls with written instructions that matched the urgency of a military commander. *Do your dishes! Take your shoes off! Take Charley's shit to the dump, not the garage!*)

After tucking him in after a 4:00 a.m. trip to the bathroom, I noticed Dad's eyes watering.

"Dad, we're going to fight this," I told him, trying to look strong.

"Mitch, you don't understand," he said, pointing at the family photos Mom had taped to the walls. "You kids look *nothing* like me ... Do you think Mom screwed the mailman?"

Sounds of His Soul
April 2020

Norman ended the call after his sister said goodnight, returning his gaze to his living-room television. As he flipped between an evening newscast and a rerun episode of *The Big Bang Theory*, his mind replayed the recent phone chat with Arlene. It was about another "big bleed in the toilet bowl."

Norman asked for Harvey's vitals and reassured his younger sister that there was no need to worry for the time being. He also said that if Harvey lost any more blood, he should be taken to the hospital again, and offered to make some calls to see which of the GTA's hospital emergency departments was the least busy.

A physician in the emergency department at Credit Valley Hospital, he took his frontline obligations seriously, reporting to duty for eight-hour shifts.

Uncle Norman, along with Daniel, Uncle Howie, and Uncle Earl, had been closely analyzing Harvey's bloodwork results from Sunnybrook and knew how fast-growing this mutation of melanoma was. He was spending hours each day researching immunotherapy and possible clinical trials, reading case after case, medication review after medication review. The torrent of information was as overwhelming as it was unproductive. And that's what made it all such a crippling burden: no matter what he learned or considered, he was fundamentally helpless in a tragedy beyond his reach. He had felt like this before.

Norman had lost his father, Buddy, to cancer, a couple decades prior. He had stayed by his father's side throughout his decline, watching his body deteriorate. He slept next to him on the hospital bed, having long chats about life and death, discussing in hushed tones the meaningful and meaningless victories of a good life beneath the beeps and hums of surrounding hospital machines. Buddy had told him to "take care of the family" days before his last breath. Norman promised he would.

After Buddy died, Norman wrote a poem, titled "My Father." "In the quietness of my thoughts, there are the sounds of his soul," it went. "His quiet spirit evokes serenity, and his loud fatherly affection gives me the strength to go on."

In all his social advocacy and emergency shifts, the memory of his father was there, pushing him to do good in the world. But now there was a wall standing between him and where he needed to be, and he wasn't sure if he should break through it.

Norman desperately wanted to go into our house and help Harvey, to care for him in-person instead of on the phone. But he didn't know if it would be safe or responsible. On the living-room TV, CBC's the *National* had been showing the latest number of fatalities from the virus. Tomorrow, he'd report to Credit Valley. His cycle of exposure would continue, trapping him in this inner conflict, splitting the bridge between professional duty and family obligation.

Norman glanced at a shelf across the couch. There was a photo of Buddy and him wearing jean jackets, smiling big. The image showed a father and son glowing with companionship and mutual respect. All these years later since it was taken, even as a sixty-two-year-old man, Norman simply missed his dad.

Sucking in air, he pointed the remote and lowered the TV's volume, attempting to tune into the quietness of his thoughts.

Suffer in Hope
April 2020

As I sat on a picnic bench next to the Sunnybrook east parking lot, under a cloudy sky, my thumbs hovered over my iPhone notepad. As I waited for Dad to complete his first treatment, I was struck with complicated relief that I was hoping to articulate through words on my screen.

I understood that immunotherapy might not be effective with Dad's type of cancer, and the long list of potential side effects had been cycling mercilessly through my mind. But every moment before this had been about maximizing his comfort. Now, something was being done to minimize the spread. I breathed in and out, and, as I often do, tried to find refuge in my words.

"I know he might enter the car feeling worse than when he left it," I wrote. "But just knowing that this new pain could be a symptom of progress, instead of a mere indication of his demise, fills me with steady optimism. I know that false hope, clinging onto a specific outcome, can be a dangerous ordeal; it can send you spiralling into disappointment and anguish. But the hope of doing something, of taking matters into our hands, of refusing to remain completely helpless, endows me with gratitude, even clarity. It makes this nightmare a little easier to manage.

"How many moments in life hinge on the promise of a better future? How many minutes are ignited by the artificial glow of tomorrow's opportunity? What does it mean to be thankful, right now, regardless of — or, in spite of — impending darkness? No clue.

"But I think the best hope is not about expectation. I think it's about choosing to be in control of your own fear. Being hopeful is not about what may happen down the line, but what is happening as you walk along it.

"I would rather suffer in hope than be comfortably hopeless."

❀

Eventually, Dad called me to say he'd be another twenty minutes. He had to sit for hours as he was injected with his immunotherapy medications. His tiredness was apparent in the gravelly quality of his voice. I told him there was no rush.

"I'm not Russian … I'm Canadian," he said.

I laughed at the joke I've heard a hundred times.

"You're the best, Dad," I said.

"You've been waiting for me for hours," he replied. "I'm not the best dad. Not even close. But one day, you'll be."

The Universal Language
May 2020

Dad's clothes looked baggy as he sat at the backyard table under the overcast sky. His outgrown hair rippled in the breeze as Earl and Louise, masked and a good distance apart, sat before him.

Louise noticed her brother's weight loss first. (She had been repeatedly dropping off food that might appeal to him: cherry pie baked by Uncle Howie; brisket slow cooked by her oldest son, Sandon; cheesecake made by Daniel.) Dad's skin looked waxier, and the whites of his eyes were slightly yellow. But besides these physical differences, he seemed himself. He cracked jokes about Trump, the virus, and the stock market — topics they'd cover if nothing was wrong. The word *cancer* wasn't mentioned.

"So, I heard the Corona beer brand is suffering because of their name, and I have the perfect solution after Trump's recent press conference ... they just gotta change the label to say hydroxy-chlorine."

Laughter.

"Hydroxychloroquine," Earl corrected.

"Yeah, that's what I said."

As sunlight beamed between parting clouds, Louise remembered seeing her brother in a hospital wing all those years ago, the day he was hit by a car when he was eleven years old. Forever etched in her memory was that forced smile on his young face, the subtle facial expression intended to put his siblings at ease. It was the same smile on her brother's face now, noticeable even with a mask.

As Dad lowered that mask and sipped his supplement drink, his lips wrapped around a plastic straw jammed into what looked like a juice box, he looked small and fragile, like a heavier wind could knock him off his seat.

Eventually, Dad's siblings waved goodbye and were replaced by Louise's sons: Daniel and his brother Sandon. Matt, Louise's middle son in Ottawa, FaceTimed in, and his son, Benjamin, waved enthusiastically on the pixelated screen. Then came Uncle Norman and his wife, Iris. Each visit was time-limited — everyone would've stayed longer if they could.

Dad took every opportunity possible to lighten the mood with his humour. After learning that his nephew Sandon had recently damaged his laptop by spilling a bowl of Fruit Loops and milk over the keyboard, Dad texted him the following message in all caps, and read it out loud for his visitors.

> THIS IS AN URGENT MESSAGE FROM KELLOGG'S! WE ARE RECALLING OUR FRUIT LOOPS PRODUCT. CUSTOMERS HAVE COMPLAINED ABOUT THE LOOPS JUMPING OFF THE SPOON AND ONTO COMPUTERS. IF THIS HAS HAPPENED TO YOU, YOU MIGHT BE ELIGIBLE FOR SUBSTANTIAL COMPENSATION.

I remember laughing at this as my eyes teared, hit with a sudden surge of fear. What, I wondered, would life be like without his singular sense of humour?

✻

At the end of the day, while I interviewed him about the family visits, Dad repeatedly expressed his gratitude for the presence of his loved ones, whether that presence was from close or afar.

"I'm getting a tremendous amount of support," he said, sitting up on his mattress, his hazel eyes dazed from morphine.

"Does it bother you that you couldn't hug anyone?" I asked.

Physical embraces had always been in his lexicon of family communication. He nodded. "When you have a serious diagnosis, you want to be as optimistic as possible, but you also want to have a sense of touch.... Hugs are like the universal language for saying, 'You're gonna be okay.'"

Thanks to a quick Google search, I discovered that psychologists and neuroscientists who have been researching the effects of hugs agree with the sentiment. The oxytocin-endorsing gesture has been proven to build a sense of security during uncertain times, and numerous studies with terminally ill patients have suggested that physical affection can help ease anxieties about dying.

The word *hug* is derived from the Saxon and Teutonic words *hog* or *hagen*, which translates as "being tender of and embracing."[2] The word *embrace* has a Latin origin — *brace*, deriving from the word *braccia*, which, in the combination *braccia collo circumdare* means "put one's arm around."[3] (I Googled

---

2 Friedrich Kluge, *An Etymological Dictionary of the German Language*, 11th ed., trans. Alfred Götze (Berlin: Walter de Gruyter, 1930).

3 Lena M. Forsell and Jan A. Åström, "Meanings of Hugging: From Greeting Behavior to Touching Implications," *Comprehensive Psychology* 1, no. 13 (January 2012).

this also.) The simplicity of that action, of "putting one's arm around," is perhaps the most fundamental and repeated reassurance of human history.

Dad and I would always do this thing, whenever I'd come home after a while away, to make Charley jealous. We'd hug each other in front of the attention-hungry goldendoodle, and he'd start pressing his nose against our legs. Then it would turn into a sort of competitive dance, where Dad, still hugging me, would try to twist my back around, and I'd try to twist his, and whoever's back was closer to Charley would feel two paws scratching for affection.

I like to think about it like this. Throughout millions of years of heartbreak and celebration, of triumph and failure, of hellos and goodbyes, the emotional affirmation of a physical embrace has remained the most continuous mode of bonding and healing in the sprawling narrative of *Homo sapiens* connection.

This universal language is encoded in our DNA, so much so that whatever pain we endure, whatever loss or turmoil or darkness we encounter, a hug can, somehow, make us feel a little better.

It did when I learned my good friend died in a motorcycle accident, when a group of weeping fraternity brothers engulfed each other in suffocating, spine-squeezing bear hugs well into the winter night.

It did in February 1996, when Mom's father died and Dad hugged her gently, offering endless support, promising her that he'd help her through the pain.

And the universal language was there yet again as I lay on the floor next to Dad's bed after his day of backyard visits. The two of us were watching *Step Brothers* on Netflix when Steph opened the door and peeked in. "Dad … can I hug you?" she asked in the glow of the hallway light, her small face no longer masked.

"Of course," Dad said, and I paused the movie.

He struggled to sit up, and my sister walked over. She bent down and wrapped her arms around him. He hugged her back, closing his eyes. Steph held back tears as she rested her head on his chest, staying in that embrace for a long moment.

Whether you're hugging your dog, friend, sibling, spouse, or father, the universal language remains a complex system of communication that can say everything you might need to say in one gesture. Because in that moment of embrace, with two stomachs rising and falling, and two hearts beating to the rhythm of an uncertain future, everything is somehow okay.

Part Three:
The Ground Beneath You

"How Bad Is It?"
May 3, 2020

While grocery shopping, Mom called me to ask how Dad was doing.

"I'm giving him another morphine," I said. "He's in a lot of pain."

"How bad is it?"

"I played Shakira, and he didn't even dance."

"Oh, *fuck*!"

Big Mac Moments
May 4, 2020

Mike and I walked slowly through the neighbourhood, enjoying the warmth of early spring sunshine. "I remember I smoked a lot of weed," he said as we cut through a park of yellowed grass. "But writing sounds like much more productive therapy."

Mike — one of my good friends and former university roommates — had lost his mother to cancer a few years ago. Talking to someone who had experienced what I was going through was both comforting and unsettling. A part of me didn't want to totally accept that this was real, and talking to Mike, who knew just how real this all was, made what was happening impossible to ignore. But it was also a little easier to accept. He, after all, was still standing. Grief hadn't swallowed him whole.

After telling him about the journal I'd been keeping every day, I asked Mike questions about what to anticipate, understanding that every cancer case is different and believing that nothing he said could make me feel better. But something did.

He told me a story about a day with his mother after her second round of targeted radiation on a metastasized brain tumour. "At this point, my mom was really close to the end and was losing her ability to talk and move," he said. We passed an elementary public school, with a couple kids dribbling a ball before a crooked basketball net.

"We had already begun to accept that she was gone. But the day after her radiation treatment, I went to the kitchen to grab a sandwich. My mom was sitting on the couch. And the moment she saw me, she perked up with wide eyes, and was like, 'Hi, Mike!'"

He stopped walking, his eyes wide with the memory. "Man, I dropped my sandwich. She seemed completely okay. I was like, 'Hey Mom! I can't believe — How are you feeling?' She looked at me with a big smile. 'Starving. Want to go to McDonald's? I *really* want a Big Mac.' I was like, 'Yeah! Of course, Mom!' So, I got in the car that evening and drove to the nearest McDonald's drive-thru and got Big Macs. I brought them back home and the two of us ate them together. It was weird because in that small moment, eating those burgers, it was like everything was normal." Mike crossed his arms as we continued down the sidewalk, a slight breeze rolling against us. "I'll never forget that Big Mac."

He told me his mother died a couple weeks after, but that wasn't the point.

When you're losing someone a little more every day, you find yourself hanging on to any glimmer, any minute of having them back. You find yourself deeply thankful for the simple moments — the moments where the person you'll soon lose isn't yet gone.

Mike and I decided to call these in-between glimmers of return "Big Mac Moments."

And I made a promise to myself that I'd appreciate every one to come.

The Story of the Pirates
May 4, 2020

I opened up an envelope and pulled out a blue sheet of construction paper that was plastered with orange and purple Crayon. A child's drawing of a floating pirate ship — it wasn't obvious at first, but we got confirmation from the artist that that's what it was. (Certain strokes of the Crayons more resembled an abstract painting you'd find in a museum of postmodernist art.) On the other side was a story, handwritten by Aunt Louise's son Matthew but first told and conceived by his four-year-old, Benjamin.

With all of us in our pyjamas — Steph, Mom, and me lounging on the carpet, and Dad on the twin bed — I read out the story. Steph filmed it so the distinguished young author could witness the reading.

The two-paragraph tale, appropriately titled "The Story of the Pirates," was about a group of pirates who were camping in the woods. At a certain point, a hockey game against Captain Hook began. (Whether this was the original crocodile-fearing pirate from Never Never Land or an entirely different villain was not really determined.) It ended with Benjamin himself flying in on a rocket and winning the game, defeating the pirate once and for all.

As I read, I made sure to pause for effect, and raised my voice for the climatic ending. ("So ... the pirates ... could play hockey again. The ... end," I intoned, trying my best to channel my inner Morgan Freeman.)

After I finished, and before Steph ended the recording to send the video to Matt, we all erupted into applause. "What a beautiful story!" Dad called, despite being dazed from his morphine and weaving out of sleep halfway.

Dad always showed exaggerated enthusiasm for the stories I wrote growing up — many of them were far less coherent than Benjamin's. He'd read my fictional rambles over and over again, telling me often how much he loved this character or that ending. He'd listen to my impassioned readings during long car rides, often interrupting to ask that I repeat a paragraph. "Just that line before … say that again? No, the other one! After that! Ya! That's brilliant! *Fucking* brilliant!"

It instilled in me a sense of confidence that stuck with me, a self-assurance that is rare in young writers. He told me he believed in me so often that I began to believe in myself. As my journalism career began to bud, he was always ready to drop everything to read one of my student newspaper articles. He'd brag about my work to his colleagues in his office, or at dinners with family friends when the conversational topic was nowhere near the accomplishments of their kids. Often, he'd look me in the eye late at night, as we'd walk Charley in our suburban neighbourhood, and say things like, "It's impossible for me to be more proud of you than I already am."

Gazing at the Crayon illustration of a pirate ship, I remembered a day Dad visited me when I was in my third year of my undergraduate program. We sat at a local pub, a sports game flashing on surrounding televisions, a couple of dartboards and movie posters decorating the walls. I was nineteen — finally of legal drinking age — and sipping a pint of Rickard's Red as Dad furiously thumbed away on his cellphone. Steaming with stress, he was completely occupied by work emails for the first twenty minutes of us sitting down. It was ironic, I thought, that he would drive any distance to be with me, but once he was here, he wasn't. Sometimes his own law firm held him hostage, like he was the warden of his own prison.

I ordered nachos and gulped beer, increasingly annoyed by Dad's lack of presence. I wasn't perfect myself — there had been countless occasions when he would call me, but I was too occupied with the melodramas of a university student to give him much attention. On this day, though, something happened that snapped Dad out of his work-obsessed trance. An email caught his focus. "Meet Benjamin" was the subject line; attached was a picture of a newborn baby, wrapped in a blue blanket.

The email was from Aunt Louise, who wrote that the delivery went well and that we now had a beautiful little boy in the family.

Now a great-uncle, Dad put his phone down and looked at me with tear-glazed eyes. "It's a boy," he said, his voice cracking.

He turned off his phone and ordered another beer, as if the weight of the joyous occasion had pulled him out of his stressful vortex, the birth of a new family member offering him solace and oxygen in his suffocating, email-trapping hell.

For the rest of the day, he was back. It served as a reminder that family was Dad's saving grace. It was then, and it would be now.

After Dad dozed off to sleep, I taped Benjamin's story and drawing onto the wall — above a photo of Steph and me as little kids.

Life Is a Series of Compromises
May 7, 2020

After someone dies, it's common for those enduring loss to compile lists of memories, to use words on a page to cement the joys of a loved one's previous presence. Writing about the people we have lost, as I did for Gaby's sister, is a natural human endeavour, a therapeutic affirmation that allows us to hang on to a past that has otherwise slipped beyond our grasp.

It's less common, however, to compile such lists of memories when the person you'll lose is still alive to reminisce and engage with. My sister, in this way, was a few steps ahead.

Late one night, Steph sat on the carpet next to Dad's bed, holding a journal with point form notes jotted on the open pages. "I wanted to write down some of my favourite memories with you," she said. "So, I've been writing one down each night before I go to bed."

She read out the long list — the two of them going for sushi on nights Mom played mah-jong with her friends; Dad's surprise visits to her university when she was pursuing her undergraduate degree; swim races in pools on vacation; playing charades during sunsets; long talks during early morning drives to work; and so on. (She also apologized for any of her angsty-teenage tantrums aimed at him when she was growing up.) The two of them stayed up late, laughing and smiling in the warm glow of recollection.

But eventually the conversation veered toward the other man Steph loved.

"What I really want you to do," Dad said, "is spend some time with Ryan. For one or two days, if you could spend a little time with him … I think that would be a nice compromise." He sat up a little and turned his head toward her on his pillow. "Life," he said, "is a series of compromises."

He told her it's not about picking sides as much as it's about choosing to participate in the inevitable struggles life throws at you. "Giving up when things get hard. That's what you want to avoid."

"Are you sure it's okay if I see him?"

"I'm not dying tomorrow," he said. The attempt at humour didn't land with Steph; her eyes blinked with tears.

"I love you, Dad," Steph said.

"I love you more," he replied tiredly. "And don't argue."

Kiss Me Arse
May 8, 2020

"How *ye* doin', *dear*?" Mom called, checking on Dad after dinner one night, as Steph and I sat on the carpet next to his bed. She was from Sydney, Nova Scotia, and often threw on a thickly exaggerated Cape Breton accent for the family's entertainment.

Speaking the few words Dad was able to muster with slightly competent imitation, he would always reply, "What's yer fadder's name?"

"My fadder's name was Buddy, what's it to you?" Mom said. "What's he gettin' at, eh, kids?"

"Kiss me arse," Dad called, switching up his typical response.

Mom pointed a finger. "Listen, we at Cape Breton arr quaaaality … *Yoo* people up *deer* in *Maaaa*-tawa think it's all great down by da *Maaaa*-tawa River where it's all *polloooooted*. Well, ma folks and me're right near da Atlantic Ocean … and we gat fresh Atlantic salmon over deer!"

"Polloooooted?" Dad called. "What's da heck's *polloooooooted*?"

"You know, what causes all dem dead fish?" Mom replied.

"Just cuz it's a smaller river don't mean it's *polloooooted*," Dad called back. Then: "What's yer fadder's name?"

"I just toll ya, dammit!"

Banter like this would often weave in and out of conversations.

Eventually, after the accents dropped, Steph and I left the room, and Mom and Dad reminisced about their years of marriage and starting a family together. They talked about the early days — swim school, dance recitals, hockey tournaments, all the chaos of a past that flashed by too quickly.

"Do you remember that visitor's day at Mitchell's first summer at camp, when we found out he somehow lost all his underwear?" Mom asked with a giggle.

"We spent half the day looking for boxers in Huntsville!"

"Socks, too! He didn't do his laundry the whole summer!"

"Half the camp's lost and found was his!"

Riding the wave of memories, they laughed freely, and after their laughter faded, Dad talked about how happy he was to have the whole family living under the same roof for the first time in a decade, how his illness and the pandemic had brought us all closer together. "It's all just … so special," he said, his words slow and heavy, his eyes glancing at the photos on surrounding walls.

In recent weeks, Arlene had noticed a change in her husband besides his physical deterioration. Over more than thirty years of marriage, the husband who had stood by her side was always extremely caring and devoted to family, but there were times when he was so consumed by his legal work that he lacked presence at the dinner table, or as they both brushed their teeth and she asked him about his day.

She had learned to accept that this was who he was, that her husband often preferred to keep his emotions to himself. But since his diagnosis, and since Steph and I had moved back to the house, she now felt that he was more present, more grounded and open than when he was healthy. She wondered if it went both ways: Was she now more attentive than before? Was she a more present wife in sickness than in health?

Arlene glanced at one of their wedding photos mounted on the wall, to the right of the bed. Two small-town kids, with big smiles and big hopes, looked back at her — Harvey wearing a tux, her in a white, clunky, shoulder-padded wedding gown. Her eyes fell to the other photos on the wall — small faces smudged with birthday cake, flaunted Halloween costumes, Sunday-morning pyjamas, grass-stained soccer jerseys. Images of family bound by love and joy. *We did good*, she thought.

"What do you think is the most important value we've instilled in our children?" Arlene asked, kneeling before his bed.

"Resilience," he responded.

"Resilience," she echoed. "I agree."

Arlene thought about how resilient her husband was, how resilient their family was. But she knew the definition of resilience — the capacity to recover quickly from difficulties, or a substance's ability to return to its original form or shape — didn't completely apply to her, because she believed that after losing Harvey, after enduring the hardships of grief, she would take on a different shape entirely. So much of who she was was linked to her husband, so much of her original form was attached to that prior life they laughed about. Whatever she'd become next, she would be something different. And she wasn't sure how different she'd be.

"What's your number?" she asked him, noticing he seemed physically uncomfortable.

She was referring to his pain level, the one-to-ten metric for determining morphine timing, but Harvey, in a lazy attempt at humour, said his phone number instead.

Smiling, Arlene rolled her eyes. "Kiss me arse."

The Ground Beneath You
May 10, 2020

"I wonder if it's easier to cry for someone you aren't that close with," I said, as Sam and I ambled through the neighbourhood one night, clouds of marijuana drifting from our joints. I took a long toke and coughed lightly, exhaling a plume of smoke into the cool air. The skunky scent followed us along, blending with the spring aroma of the quiet suburban night.

"Crying for someone who's such a major part of your life seems too … overbearing," I continued. "Your body doesn't know how to function without that person in your life; your mind rejects the possibility of their absence…. Crying almost seems like a waste of time. How could that person not be here? That person is the ground beneath your feet. Without the ground, you'll never stop falling …"

Sam patiently listened to my rant as we jaywalked across an empty street, beneath the white glow of a few streetlights. He was that friend who was always there for you, the guy who would drop everything to be by your side when shit hit the fan. Along with the joints, he had brought me a copy of *Tuesdays with Morrie*, the famous 1997 bestseller by Mitch Albom.

It was one of my favourite books, and I had lost my own copy a couple years ago. After I told Sam this, he was quick to order a new one and drop it off. The relevance of the story about a journalist (with the same first name) interviewing a dying man was achingly apparent.

When I first began interviewing Dad, a part of me was hoping the exchange would be similar, that Dad's wisdom would be as poignant and accessible as Morrie Schwartz's, the dying man in Albom's book — he expounds about his philosophy on living a meaningful life and embracing death in all its horrific stages. My dad, for the most part, didn't match Morrie's eloquence. (Most of us don't.) Dad wasn't a sociology professor, had never published books about social dichotomy, and his life convictions weren't as distilled and servable as those presented by Morrie, who deployed his thoughts with the organization and structure of a lecture delivered in a senior-level college course.

But Dad *did* know what it was like to grieve, to be parentless and helpless in an unforgiving world — to draw optimism despite treacherous and soul-crushing circumstances. I knew there was a reservoir of fossilized wisdom deep beyond his hardened surface. I just didn't know if I could excavate it before it was too late.

I hadn't cried in weeks, and I wasn't sure why. I figured it was a classic case of journalistic compartmentalization, of distancing myself from the story unfolding around me, as if what was happening to my family was some fuzzy abstraction I was looking at from afar instead of from within. I felt numb. Disconnected. And, speaking to Sam, I was trying to unpack why.

"Maybe it's just too difficult to mourn something you feel that you can't live without," I said, stepping over some potholes on the moonlit street, both of us forgetting the sidewalk and moving down the middle of a car lane. "It's too difficult to accept that it's possible for that person to really be gone. You prefer living in denial. And when you're in denial, there's no need to cry, because there's nothing that's missing.... You still have the ground beneath you."

"That makes a lot of sense," Sam said, exhaling a cloud. "But, whatever the reason, I think it's okay that you're not crying.... You have to give yourself permission to feel however you're feeling."

Sam's response showed he detected some sort of guilt. I realized he was spot on. Deep down, I had been feeling *guilty* for not crying.

If I loved my dad so much, why wasn't I bawling my eyes out every second? Why wasn't I welling with emotion as I noticed his fragile body deteriorating? It made me guilty and angry, alienated from the unfazed soldier I had turned into. I had become so adept at swallowing my emotions that, it seemed, I had lost access to them.

I told Sam about the conversation I had had with Mike recently — the Big Mac Moments I'd been journaling about, those in-between glimmers of return that can momentarily brighten the darkness of dying and loss. Always a loyal supporter of my journalistic work, Sam told me to keep writing and to keep my eyes open. "I think those moments could happen anytime," he said.

After the joints were killed, we waved goodbye and walked our separate ways. It was almost two in the morning when I finally arrived home.

I later described what happened next in an essay published in a newspaper: "I disabled the alarm, pulled off my shoes, and sprayed a little Lysol on my sweatshirt. Then I tiptoed out of the laundry room like I always used to when I'd come home late and didn't want to wake anyone from one of the many groaning floorboards."

Dad had been getting weaker and more dependent every day, and the simple task of walking down the hall was becoming incredibly difficult. But on this night, such difficulty wouldn't stop him.

Groaning, he threw off his covers and struggled to sit up. The moment his legs thumped against the carpet, nausea surged through him. He sucked in some air, gripped the bed's headrest, and pulled himself onto his feet.

Walking used to be easier, he remembered, as he shimmied forward, using the upstairs banister for balance, his blurry eyes steadily focused on the shadowed, hardwood floor. His legs felt weaker than ever; when he tried to lift them, it felt like invisible ankle weights were strapped to each foot.

Well, now I'm really *a useless schmuck*, declared his endlessly self-deprecating internal monologue as he moved forward at snail-speed. The room at the end of the hall seemed far away. His stomach growled with indigestion, bubbling and groaning with occasional pangs of pain. Ignoring it, he put one foot in front of the other. Dizziness didn't matter. More nausea ... so what? *My son needs me.*

He had been lying restlessly, trying not to let his thoughts and fears get the best of him. Weaving in and out of sleep, he kept focusing on the photos he was able to see in the darkened room, nothing but the soft light of the TV's clock illuminating the smiling faces taped to the walls. He knew that soon enough he would need to go to the bathroom but didn't want to wake Steph — who would call out to him to make sure he was okay. He hated being the burden he had become. He only wanted to be there for his kids, to keep them safe and protected, to do what he'd always done. He didn't want them to worry. That was always *his* job.

And so, after hearing my bedroom door close around two in the morning, there he was, putting one foot in front of the other, making a trip down the hall he hadn't done alone in days, being the father he'd always been.

He made it to the end and extended his arm to open the door. But the moment he did, that door swung open. He saw my concerned face.

"I just wanted to make sure you were home safe," Dad said, slightly out of breath, sounding almost apologetic for intruding.

After a moment of registration, I wrapped my arms around him, hugging him tight.

Dad's frail arms squeezed me back, his stomach — pressed against mine — as supportive as the ground beneath my feet. Thankful for the Big Mac Moment, my eyes began to well.

Favourite Colour
May 13, 2020

Lying on the floor next to his bed after watching the last episode of *Tiger King*, I turned on my iPhone audio recorder and interviewed Dad again.

Questions about his mother or father seemed to be too much for him, so I settled for simpler questions that I didn't know the answer to, like how old he was when he had his first kiss, and what his favourite colour was. After I asked that last one, he didn't answer and seemed to have fallen back asleep. But eventually he said, "Charcoal grey."

"Like the colour of your old Audi?" I asked.

"Yeah."

It was in that car that he drove me to hockey practice, Steph to dance competitions, Mom to dinner dates with friends. That car was the vehicle of his former life, and it was the car he had sold shortly before the pandemic, weeks before we realized he was sick. A new black Sonata sat in our garage in its place, barely used, with the new car smell lingering on its leather seats. (He was quick to purchase it after seeing its Super Bowl commercial with Amy Poehler and Chris Evans. "It's a smawt pawck!" he'd call, summoning his best Boston accent.)

Knowing it was time for my questions to graduate beyond middle-school sleepover territory, I decided to dive deep.

"Are you afraid of dying?"

He thought about it for a while, breathing slowly. "I don't think so," he said. "I'm only afraid of not being with my family anymore.... The care you all have shown me ... it makes it difficult to be afraid. All I can think about is how lucky I am to have people that will do whatever it takes to make me comfortable. Sometimes at night, when I'm alone with my thoughts, I get a little scared. But then, next thing I know, you or Steph or Mom checks on me, and the gratitude I have for that is so much stronger than my fear." After saying this, he struggled to sit up, having to go to the bathroom again.

"Besides, the fight's not over yet."

Red Light
May 25, 2020

Late one night, Dad's increased liver enzymes led to some delirium. He began trying to explain something but was making little sense. Incoherent sentences, broken by laboured breaths, had us on high alert.

A nurse on the phone suggested that we take him to Sunnybrook. They would admit him for a couple of nights and run some tests. His pain had been steadily increasing every day. Something was definitely wrong. Whatever was happening was very different from what Dad had experienced before. Mom packed an overnight bag, and he and I hopped in the car.

After dropping him off, driving alone down the dark street, I tried to slow my breathing and calm my fears. I was losing him a little more every day, and I was afraid that the man I dropped off would not be the same one I'd pick up.

What scared me the most, even more than the unanticipated speed of his physical deterioration, was the delirium. I was afraid of him losing his mind. Of *me* losing his mind. He was finally more vulnerable, more accessible, than he'd ever been, and I was afraid of losing that before I was ready. There were so many questions I still needed to ask him. So many stories I needed to uncover.

A motorcycle roared past my car in the right lane, and my chest constricted. I gripped the wheel tighter. Breathing out, I hit play on the sound system hooked up to my iPhone, and "Elias" came on. A few seconds in, I turned it off and slammed the steering wheel with my palm, a wave of emotion and thoughts bursting through my heart and brain.

Dad had always wielded unwavering optimism. He was a man armoured by unjustified positivity. And for so long, I felt I should be wearing the same armour. But as the tires rolled over the smooth road that night, with nothing but the quietness of the AC filling the car and the light hiss of wind against the windshield, I took that armour off … and began to scream.

I yelled with the fury exploding inside me, anger so deep that it blurred my vision. Loud, shrill noises burst from my trembling mouth between gasping breaths. For a moment, I floored the gas on the deserted road, gunning the car.

The needle on the speedometer jumped. Streetlights flashed past. The engine rumbled; the car's frame creaked. I missed my turn but kept speeding forward. A final, thunderous shout erupted out of me.

Then, approaching a red light, I slowed the vehicle to a stop. Breathing heavily, I began to cry.

All my anger dissolved into despair, and I didn't stop weeping the rest of the way home.

The ground beneath me was crumpling. And I wasn't ready to begin my fall.

Crazy Place
May 25, 2020

"You okay?"

Norman, sitting in the staff lounge of Credit Valley Hospital's emergency department, looked up from his cellphone. His colleague Alice was looking at him through her face shield. "You've seemed distracted lately."

Norman exhaled tiredly. "It's my brother-in-law, actually," he said, his eyes falling back to one of the many texts Arlene had sent him. "The one I told you about … He's just been admitted at Sunnybrook. Might be an adverse reaction to his treatment."

"Chemo?"

"Immunotherapy."

Alice took a seat in front of him. The two emergency physicians had had a few moments of confession prior, about the difficulties of compartmentalizing the grim prognoses of their patients in their professional life. Alice had recently lost her mother to cancer. Norman had talked about losing his father decades ago. They spoke about how they see them — their mothers, their fathers, Harvey, in the faces of patients they diagnose. "Work's becoming more and more difficult to separate from life," Norman said.

Both doctors had witnessed a phenomenon that had been documented in public records since March 2020: with clinics shut down and patients unable to receive physical assessments and adequate monitoring of symptoms, there has been a significant uptick of patients coming in with advanced-stage cancer.

Norman remembered a patient he had treated recently who had been complaining about severe back pain. The sixty-year-old woman had five virtual meetings, over a span of four months, with her general practitioner to discuss her worsening suffering. After she came into the emergency room, Norman evaluated the case and decided to conduct a thorough investigation. X-rays and CT scans revealed metastasized spinal tumours.

"The worst part," Norman once said to Alice, "is not even being able to look their family in the eye as you tell them over the phone."

A nurse came in and told Norman about a patient he had been waiting on. It was a thirty-three-year-old male with a recently detected brain tumour. "Crazy place we work, eh?" he called, before leaving.

Alice only nodded.

Brave
May 26, 2020

Around ten one night, we FaceTimed Dad. He answered on his hospital bed. His dazed eyes brightened when he saw Mom, Steph, and me gathered on a mattress.

"Hey, Harv," Mom called.

"Hey, hun!" Dad said, cheerfully.

"Remember that time we went to that pop-up choir event and sang those songs?"

Dad nodded. "Of course."

"Well, I sent you a video of us singing that song by Sara Bareilles —"

Dad interrupted her, crooning a line about being brave from the chorus.

"Yup," Mom said. "We thought we'd bring some karaoke to your hospital wing. Feel free to sing along, hun."

Steph hit play on her laptop, and the song "Brave" started playing. Or, it was supposed to.

"Turn up the volume," Mom said.

"I'm trying! There's an ad!"

"Skip it!"

"It won't let me! Okay there —"

"Louder!"

"It's as loud as it goes!"

Our start delayed, we struggled to harmonize. Mom had printed off the lyrics for us, but some words were difficult to make out. So, a few seconds behind, we rushed chaotically to catch up with Sara Bareilles, tripping over notes until we arrived at the chorus. Our voices unified as we sang the lyrics about being brave enough to open your heart and mouth and having the inner faith to join them together.

"Honestly ... my farts sound better," Dad chirped over the crashing mess of a family with no musical talent.

Between bursts of child-like giggles, Steph continued the song. It was then that my sixty-seven-year-old father began making farting sounds with his mouth.

"Real mature, Harv," Mom called.

Steph kept singing, screeching like a wounded cat as she echoed Dad's favourite line.

"Dear God, please stop!" Dad called, as if her voice was causing him physical pain. "It was sweet and all, but it's *enough*!"

At that, I fell off the bed laughing.

Drink Water!
May 29, 2020

The day after he was wheeled out of the hospital, where he had been admitted for three nights, Dad put on a suit and tie and joined a pre-trial on Zoom at our kitchen table.

What the judge, his client, and opposition didn't know was that his liver enzymes were alarmingly high, that his thighs and calves were blown up like elephant legs beneath the table, and that his body was shutting down. They didn't know that he had — maybe — two weeks to live, and that he was spending four hours of his limited time advocating for his client.

In the memoir *When Breath Becomes Air*, Paul Kalanithi, a thirty-something-year-old neurosurgeon diagnosed with Stage 4 lung cancer, grapples with the demands of continuing his work as a surgeon while his body gradually fails him. Recognizing that meaning derives from serving a purpose larger than himself, Kalanithi sought such meaning in his work until he was no longer physically capable of continuing. When justifying his decision to spend much of his remaining days wearing a lab coat, gripping a scalpel, and slaving over complicated procedures that his healthier colleagues would have been equally capable of orchestrating, he considered the simple truth that moral duty has weight. "Things that have weight have gravity," he wrote. "And so the duty to bear mortal responsibility pulled me back into the operating room."

Much like Kalanithi and his surgeries, Dad found deep meaning in continuing to advocate for his client, in representing someone in need and carrying out his contractual obligations. He didn't have mortal responsibility, in the sense that people's lives weren't in his hands — at least, not in the literal way they were in Kalanithi's — but he did have an urge to help people, to use his knowledge and skill set to benefit another life.

This urge brought him back to the courtroom, albeit a virtual one. Yet, there was another weight magnetizing his efforts, a sensation hard to find once you begin wearing adult diapers: a feeling of empowerment.

Returning to his familiar domain of legal jargon and pre-trial proceedings that day, he was back to doing what he did well, feeling in control while losing his battle with an illness rendering him helpless. Maybe, even in the worst of suffering, the combined recipe of moral duty, deeper purpose, and a sense of self-sufficiency and mastery is the only antidote for accepting a future that doesn't include you.

As the pre-trial proceeded, with cross-examinations of documented evidence and a thorough assessment of witness testimonials, Mom and Steph held up paper signs that said *Drink water!* They hoisted them like cheerleaders on the side-lines of a football field.

In between light coughs, Dad casually sipped his water, ig-noring the pain in his rectum, the nausea and fatigue swirling through him as he maintained baseline focus. He was deter-mined to finish the job.

The pre-trial was a hard-hitting demonstration of my father's brilliance and acute attention to detail. The case in-volved a car accident, but it wasn't your typical rear-end col-lision. It dealt with a motorist and another car's driver who pulled out of a street parking spot before using their signal and without checking their blind spot. The motorist ended up hitting the car. As a result of the accident, he suffered serious brain injuries. Dad argued vigorously for the motorist, dis-secting the case, highlighting the timing of the signal delay, the speed of the other motorist's acceleration, the required space to effectively stop, and every minute but necessary detail of the incident. He deconstructed every moment of the accident with exhaustive but genius precision, reminding everyone who they were dealing with: that pain-in-the-ass personal injury lawyer who would stop at nothing to help his client and use the legal system for justice.

Eventually, the case was settled in his client's favour, and Dad thanked the judge, who he knew, for his many years of service. He told him that he likely wouldn't be around soon, that he was diagnosed with fast-growing cancer, and that he was thankful for everyone's time. Then he closed his laptop, ending his thirty-nine-year career on a good note.

❋

Shortly after, Louise, Earl, and much of the family visited. They had begun coming inside, wearing masks and keeping their distance. Dad, in his stand-up comedian mood, told stories and jokes. "You know, I've been doing some research on something called an 'ancient Egyptian retainer sacrifice,'" he said, leaning back on the couch. "When pharaohs were dying and they wanted their servants to join them in the afterlife, they arranged for them to be slaughtered." Dad took a sip of water. "So … you all might want to watch your backs."

It took a few seconds to register what he was implying — mostly because the darkness of the joke went far beyond his typical humour. Uncle Norman started chuckling first, his infectious, deep-belly giggles rising up, turning into coughs and heaves. "We're the servants!" he bellowed.

The moment the rest of us clued in, a massive eruption of

laughter followed, filling the living room with the auditory elixir Dad craved. He smiled with satisfaction.

❋

Humour, as uplifting as it was, quickly made way for sadness on the emotional rollercoaster each of us involved in my father's end-of-life care rode.

Later in the afternoon, I caught Uncle Earl sobbing in the laundry room, and the moment he saw me he swallowed his sadness, like I've seen my father do a hundred times. I hugged him. It was the first hug I had given to someone outside my immediate family since March.

Hours after that, Mom, Steph, Dad, and I had our last pyjama dance party.

More for the necessity of activating his atrophied muscles than inspired by the mood of the moment, Dad struggled to keep standing as he lazily threw his arms around to the music, swaying weakly, his inner underwear-flaunting rockstar unable to fully emerge.

Falling
May 31, 2020

Around two thirty in the morning, I checked on Dad after he had run to the washroom. As I tucked him in, he said he had a dream about falling. He said there was a ceiling of wires above him, one of them might've been around his neck. And it was dark and he fell and didn't know how to hang on. Then he said I caught him. He said his love for me saved him.

I told him I'd always be there to catch him when he fell.

"I know," he said, closing his eyes.

I expected a final joke, but none came.

Bumps
May 1974

The blade glided along his neck, clearing the shaving cream — and halted over the bumps. Max lowered the razor on the sink counter.

With two fingers, he felt beneath his jaw, looking into the mirror. The face of a fifty-three-year-old man, with tired, dark eyes, looked back. The stress of recent years had aged him — he could see deeper wrinkles etched into his forehead — but the bumps were something new.

Shortly afterward, the doctor confirmed they were swollen lymph nodes. Further tests led to an official diagnosis: lymphoma — cancer of the lymphatic system.

The Conskys had moved to Toronto from Mattawa eight years prior. Max and Sandra always knew that being the only Jewish family in a small town had an expiry date. It was only a matter of time until their kids would want to find Jewish partners, connect to the larger Jewish community, and immerse themselves in the life offered by a bigger city. The move was excitedly anticipated by the whole family.

But a year after moving to a nice house in Willowdale, an area in north Toronto, the doctors identified metastasizing tumours on Sandra's liver. A year of chemo and medication followed this discovery. In the summer of 1967, she died.

Earl and Louise were at sleep-away camp that summer, taking weekly buses back to Toronto, switching between two worlds: one of colour wars and cabin hopping, and one of chemo and morphine. Harvey had stayed home, wanting to be near his mother. Sandra had begun knitting Harvey a sweater but never finished it.

Life, as painful as it was, continued without her. When she was twenty-two, Louise married an emergency doctor named Howard. Earl and Harvey moved into an apartment on St. George Street. Max remarried. He continued driving back and forth to Mattawa to operate the theatre. He tried to make the most of the life he'd been given.

Then came the bumps on his neck. The diagnosis. The threat of death re-emerging, this time the threat aimed at himself. Max had been seriously sick before — he'd had a severe case of ulcerative colitis — but illness never held him back long. He was engaged in a different type of fight now. He had seen what cancer could do.

Max's kids had lost their mother only seven years earlier. He didn't want them to worry about their father — of course, they constantly did. Despite having to undergo regular chemo sessions, he continued to manage the Mattawa theatre. He took a trip to Israel with some friends. He remained a present father, being there for his kids in any way he could, never complaining about his worsening condition.

But then came a day in February 1975, about nine months after discovering those bumps in the mirror, when Max entered the hospital for a chemotherapy session and never returned home.

Nice Cheese
May 15, 2020

"Hun, if I don't make it, you need to live your life," Harvey said one night. "I hope you can find a man who will make you happy."

Arlene nodded slowly as she kneeled next to Harvey's bed, her eyes sparkling as she glanced back at that wedding photo mounted on the wall.

She had broached the topic of her being with another man in the future, knowing it was a conversation spouses should have with a dying partner. But actually hearing her husband say those words of permission filled her with a flood of emotion. Her mind travelled back to the night they met — a story Dad often told.

It was New Year's Eve, 1986, when he entered a party he wasn't invited to and first encountered a beautiful woman in a pink sweater.

She appeared next to him at the cheese table — a party space of comfort, a safe haven for someone who needed to take cover from the social anxieties of a sweaty, congested gathering of people they don't know. Noting other men competing for her time, Harvey knew he had to say something before the moment expired. He searched his mind for a suitable opening line, something clever, or funny, or insightful. He gazed at the cheese assortment on large plates.

"Uh ... nice cheese, eh?" was his chosen zinger.

Miraculously, it was enough to serve as the beginning of a conversation. (To this day, we have no idea how Arlene could have possibly followed up.) They spoke for a few minutes, covering the broad strokes. She was also from a small town, he learned. Jewish? Check. Smart? Also check. Wow, look at that smile. The daughter of a dentist.

"Call me," Harvey said at the end of that talk, over the music and surrounding chatter.

"No," Arlene said. "You call me."

Arlene would be visiting her family in Cape Breton the next day and told Harvey that she would be back in a week. He decided to play it cool, choosing to wait awhile after she arrived home before calling. He didn't want to look desperate. But he lost count of the days, forgetting when she said she'd be leaving and coming back. The second she walked back into her Toronto apartment, her phone was ringing.

"Hey ... it's Harvey ... the guy from the cheese table."

"Oh ... Harvey! Right! I'm literally just getting in now ... do you mind calling back later?"

Shit. "Yeah … no worries at all!"

Their first date went well. The conversation and wine flowed. A movie followed. A play. A first kiss. Long walks. Longer phone calls.

Arlene appreciated his sense of humour. He was self-deprecating but also goofy, like a kid who refused to fully grow up, despite the seriousness of his profession. But there was a guarded part of him also.

He had lost both of his parents before they met, and they were a topic of discussion he routinely avoided. He didn't want to let her into his pain.

Other characteristics, however, shone through, deepening their connection. She had never met someone so loyal, and supportive, and driven to do good in the world. He had an immaculate sense of fashion — an eye for detail that was as apparent in the colour of the ties he chose to wear with his suits as it was in his attention to the intricacies of a complicated case. He was intelligent, but not intimidating. Devoted, but not clingy. Independent, but not closed-off.

She noted his generosity when he would scramble for change after passing a homeless person on the street, or when his eyes would tear while he watched a newscast that covered a natural disaster ravaging the lives of helpless civilians. She loved how he treated her own mother, with respect and compassion and boxes of chocolates. Driving, it seemed, was one of his love languages, and he'd drive her to any destination, no matter the hour or distance or weather. He always put her first.

Within a year, Arlene knew she wanted to marry him.

All this time later, as she knelt before Harvey's bed, surrounded by family photos that marked the life they had built, the life that now seemed so fleeting, it amazed her that it all started at a cheese table.

"Love you, Harv," she said, squeezing his hand.

"Love you more," he said. "Don't argue."

The *Globe*
June 1, 2020

I was standing in line at a drugstore's pharmacy desk, waiting for my father's medication refill, when I got a message from a friend telling me to check the *Globe and Mail* website. "Your essay's up!"

I first wrote the story, detailing what happened the night my dad checked on me after a marijuana-infused walk, as a text to Sam. It was nothing more than my version of a Big Mac Moment I felt an urge to share as a messy and convoluted message. He immediately told me it was one of the most beautiful little anecdotes he's heard and suggested I write a longer essay about it.

When I first submitted the nine-hundred-word piece to the First Person editor of Toronto's *Globe and Mail*, one of Canada's leading newspapers, I thought it would be a while until I heard back. But Catherine, the section's editor, got back to me right away. She offered to run it on Father's Day weekend, but I had a gut feeling that would be too late.

I wanted my dad to read it in print before he was too gone — or, *actually* gone — and, after I told Catherine about this urgency, she bumped it up to the first week of June.

That story I wrote for the *Walrus* about families of health-care workers wouldn't be published for a couple months, so, after finding the link and opening it, I was now staring at my first national byline — a big moment for every journalist, but one, in this case, complicated by the emotional undercurrent of the content.

I had asked Dad for permission if I ever wanted to publish something about his cancer battle, and he gave it, without knowing much more. I hoped he'd appreciate it. I didn't love the digital headline — "Dad is dealing with a lot right now, but he still checks up on me" — because it seemed like too much of an understatement and also spoiled the conclusion of the story. (On a separate note, I also retrospectively felt like the baseball analogy I used was a little cliché.) But the accompanying illustration brought tears to my eyes.

The blue-and-black image showed a boy, with hands in his pockets, walking up a staircase, a silhouette of a larger man, presumably a father, looming over him at the top. The walls were covered in shooting stars, alive with moonlight, accentuating the shadow of the waiting dad. The boy and the father, frozen in stride, would meet halfway on that starlit staircase.

I sent an email to the illustrator, Rachel Wada, telling her how much I loved it. The next day, it was printed in the paper and distributed to millions of readers.

✦

We had set up a table in his bedroom for Dad to eat his breakfast, since the simple task of walking downstairs was becoming increasingly challenging. After we poured some meal replacement drink into a glass and placed a bowl of cut-up fruit before him, I laid out the day's issue of the *Globe*, and opened it to the First Person section.

At this point, Dad had already pieced together that I had written and published something. The essay was shared on Facebook, and the outpouring of comments and messages the whole family had been getting was hard to contain.

The headline for the printed version was much more impactful than the one online: "Always Watching Over Me." Dad read it over and over again, with a smile of pride on his face. "You're amazing," he said, and my chest felt heavy.

Afterward, Mom read him some of the comments online. Messages flooded in — one from a woman in Newfoundland, one from Winnipeg, many from Vancouver, hundreds from Toronto. Louise told us her friends had been calling her all day after reading it. Earl said his dentist read it. "Now the whole country knows how great of a father you are!" emailed one of Dad's buddies.

I also got countless messages from Facebook friends who have gone through cancer battles with loved ones — mothers, fathers, a sister. People from all over were touched by my words, relating to the pressure and turmoil of caregiving, the trials of role reversal which emerge when a family member is rendered a little more dependent.

But the joy and camaraderie of those comments and messages were disrupted by an unsettling medical update.

On the phone, Dr. Petrella told us about the unlikelihood of the treatment working given his adverse reaction. This wasn't breaking news. Looking at my dad, we knew he didn't have much time.

Being Mortal
June 4, 2020

"My friend from med school pointed me toward a promising clinical trial in the States," Daniel said as Charley sniffed grass and scouted a suitable spot to do his business. "No promises, but if we act quickly, Harvey might be eligible ..."

The whole family was visiting when Mom, Daniel, and I went for a walk to the mailbox, with Charley pulling us along.

We appreciated his optimism, but Mom and I had begun to accept the shitty cards we'd been dealt. Dad was weaker than he'd ever been, and the cancer was spreading too quickly to stop. No clinical trial was going to take someone in his condition, and, deep down, Daniel knew this.

Still, his need to help, to do something, seemed to be haunting him. He had begun reading *Being Mortal* by Atul Gawande. It's a book that argues for the benefits of accepting the inevitability of death, about how it's possible to instil meaning in the end of life. It talks about embracing the circumstances of dying rather than continually fighting to survive — a way of thinking that seems at odds with the philosophy of medicine.

Throughout the first wave of the pandemic, Daniel's emergency shifts had left him with lingering questions about end-of-life care. How do you find meaning in a life without hope? When does the need to live fully outweigh the need to live longer? How can a team of healthcare workers, trained in fixing the intricate problems that can beset the human body, learn to apply their skills to purposes beyond repair and solution? What can they do to help someone die with grace and dignity?

It was on that walk, with those questions in mind, that the idea emerged: we could utilize our family of healthcare workers to set up a hospice at home, taking a family-based approach to end-of-life care.

The Dancer
June 6, 2020

The DVD was loaded and, after one of us hit play, a thirteen-year-old Stephanie appeared on stage — the song "Popular," from the musical *Wicked*, started booming. It was another of the many old dance videos we'd been resorting to for evening entertainment, and Dad was eating it up. He marvelled at his daughter's acrobatic abilities, her ability to walk on her hands and do backflips, her precise, choreographed movements, her animated smile.

Sitting in the living room on the couch, with her thirteen-year-old self leaping around on the TV, Steph wanted to tell Dad that Ryan was the one, that they were going to get married. She wished he would be alive for the wedding, or, at the very least, a proposal. But it seemed that that wasn't going to happen anytime soon.

Steph had spent the day with Ryan, together but at a distance. They chatted about everyday things, but eventually they moved on to discussing bigger topics — what they wanted in life, their priorities, where they saw their relationship, their future. What amazed Steph the most was that, despite their physical distance, and the demands of his residency, Ryan had remained constantly available over the last couple of months. Somehow, they had grown closer. She loved him deeply and was certain she wanted to build a life with him.

After the last video, Dad played the song "Dear Mr. President" by Pink. (It was a song in one of Steph's recitals when she was twelve.) As the music ascended, Steph danced for us on the living room's wooden floor. Only it was in a way I haven't seen her dance since she was a little girl in those videos, since she had the confidence and self-assurance of a child unscathed by a harsh world.

She would tell me after that this sudden performance was meaningless, that she was merely using muscle memory. She was seemingly oblivious to the effect she had on the man with mesmerized eyes. The man who, all those years ago, would jump up in applause after each recital performance, bursting with pride, pointing a shaky camera, calling her name.

Her eyes sparkled as she reached and leaped and spun with lyrical grace. Normally, she was just joking around when she did something performative like this at home, carrying out another goofy dance routine to match her father's sporadic moves, but it seemed to me like, this time, something else was driving her. She was simultaneously younger and older — a little girl moving in a studio and a grown woman swirling, expressing the years of lived experience within her, a dancer weathered by joy and sadness.

The way she moved with improvised lyricism, it was as if she was showing her dad, and herself, that the little girl she once was, the one he took to dance recitals and competitions, the one he put show makeup on and cheered on from theatre seats, was still inside her. She'd been there all along. And, although that little girl was in pain now, she was stronger than ever.

Dad watched, enchanted, his foot, on the end of the couch, tapping to the beat, the lyrics about a president with little regard for the state of the world reverberating through the room.

As Steph danced, I thought about how time functions differently when someone you love is dying. Laughter lasts a little longer. Joy runs a little deeper. Simple things seem more spellbinding.

Amid the turmoil of pain, there is, sometimes, an air of freedom, an unrestrained expansiveness, where the future outcome that awaits does not define the moment. This is what you discover when, instead of looking forward, you find yourself looking around.

What I had around me was a list of contradictions, a series of suspended moments that do not typically coincide with misery and despair. Despite the ending creeping closer, despite the isolation of a lockdown and the darkness engulfing the globe, laughter, joy, and dancing had, somehow, filled the house of a dying man.

Blue Eyes
June 8, 2020

I was in a small hospital room with yellow fluorescent lighting illuminating my sick father. He was struggling to sit up, his legs so swollen he had to wear shorts, his breathing increasingly laboured. The task of staying upright had become painful and draining for him, and even as he rested on the recliner chair, exhaustion was overwhelming him, sucking every ounce of his being into an internal vacuum, that black hole that devoured a bigger piece of him every day.

I had emailed Dr. Petrella a week prior, anticipating the possibility of bad news, asking if I could be by my father's side if he would be told that all hope had expired. She emailed me back, saying the decision would be up to the hospital administrators. Shortly after, I got approval, and I told Dad they had lifted the restrictions so every patient could be accompanied by one visitor. This was a lie. Hopeless circumstances had enabled the arrangement, but I wasn't ready to banish his hope by explaining this. That would be someone else's task.

Eventually, Dr. Petrella walked in. I had only heard her voice on the phone, and it was startling to see her in person. It struck me that the commander of this cancer battle, our first line of defence and beacon of hope, was just a person holding a clipboard.

"Hi, Harvey, how are you doing today?" Dr. Petrella said, after introducing herself to me.

She didn't waste time and told us what she knew. Her words were professional, precise. She explained that the blood-work didn't look good. That the metastasization had spread further. That things were irreversibly bad. The sound of her voice was disarming and matter-of-fact, honest and direct. But her blue eyes beneath her face shield told a different story. They were with me, they shared my pain, they extended her sympathy, her compassion, her sorrow.

It was this moment of eye contact that suddenly made me aware of one of the pandemic's biggest consequences: not only did we now have to face uncertainty, shutdowns, the fear of our old world crumbling, we also had to face the loss of the communication that occurs beyond words shaped by lips, beyond letters formed by markings on a page or pixels on a screen, the loss of the expression that a set of eyes can articulate as they look into another pair, as they share the weight of a moment, as they say, with empathetic feeling, "I'm sorry for your pain."

Dr. Petrella patted Dad's swollen leg with a latex-gloved hand. "I'm sorry," she said, her voice a little softer. "All we can do now is make you comfortable. And it seems like you have an amazing family that will do everything they can to make that happen."

❖

After Dr. Petrella answered all our questions, I pushed Dad in his wheelchair to the elevator down the hall. He told me to thumb the down button, believing that was the way to the exit and parking lot. I knew we needed to go up and connect to a different elevator because of the wheelchair. "No, Dad. We need to go up first," I said.

"No, we need to go down," he said.

"Dad … it's up. I *know* we need to go up."

"I said, *Hit down*!"

"Dad —"

"Hit *down*!" he shouted, turning a few heads.

"It's *up*!" I barked back.

Pretty ridiculous, right? A fight about the direction of an elevator immediately after being told time was up. An argument about nothing when everything was crashing down. I guess his outburst made me angry. But there was more: his stubbornness at that moment, and also the stubbornness that I felt, brought us here in the first place — the stubbornness that refused to believe that the pain in his ass that turned out to be a deadly tumour was anything but harmless hemorrhoids. The same stubbornness that stopped him from checking in with himself, eating right, exercising, meditating, being healthy. Sure, he went to spin classes every couple weeks and ate my mother's cooking, and I knew, of course, meditation wouldn't have stopped cancer metastasization, and I realize it was irrational to believe his circumstances were within his — or anyone's — control, but I was devastated that I wouldn't have a father who would meet the woman I'd marry, and that my future children would never meet their grandfather, and I was mad that Steph wouldn't have her dad to walk her down the aisle, and that Mom would never grow old with her husband, and, mostly, I was mad that I couldn't stop this, and I was mad that he didn't think to before it was too late.

The up-elevator arrived and, swallowing my anger, I walked us in. "I love you, Dad," I said, on the verge of tears. "But we need to go up."

New Bubble
June 8, 2020

Dad slept upstairs as the rules of the pandemic dissolved in our house: my whole family hugged and cried into each other's shoulders. Charley, detecting our sadness, pressed his muzzle against our legs.

Our despair fuelled a plan. We would become a newly formed bubble, merging our efforts, heightening our combined support, and squeezing out the most meaning we possibly could in Dad's final days — however many he still had.

We'd create a hospice at home, one that built on the foundation of love and togetherness that we had already laid. We'd keep the door open at all hours and begin a twenty-four-hour-care operation. The medical expertise of our family would take a different approach to healthcare. They'd help my father die with dignity, surrounding him with love until his very last breath. I looked around at our team, those who would join us for the final hours of a battle we would not win. It was good company to have.

But our team would include someone else, an unofficial member of the family. As the sun dipped over the horizon, Steph's boyfriend, Ryan, stepped through the front door of our house. Then, for the first time in months, he gave her a hug.

Our army was then complete.

Part Four: Morphine and Honey

Proof
June 2020

"Do you believe in God?" I asked Dad late one night as I sat on the carpet next to his bed, listening to his strenuous breathing. He was not a religious man.

Friends and relatives who had read my article in the *Globe* had been messaging me that they're "praying for him." They were telling me that he was in their prayers. That their thoughts and prayers were with my family. The word *pray* dominated my incoming messages. It felt like I was walking by one of those agents of God with a megaphone on a busy street corner preaching about the Lord and Saviour and the salvation that could only come through religious devotion.

I realized these were the typical expressions deployed during hopeless situations like this, language often used more out of custom than belief. But it got me thinking about a conversation Dad and I haven't yet had: a talk about the dude upstairs.

Belief in God, for many people, is a hazy, avoided topic. We may indulge in religious rituals, participate in dressed-up customs and annual holidays, but rarely do we genuinely engage in a serious conversation about religion or the divine, even in our own families. At least, it's not a conversation many people openly have. Dad said prayers on Friday nights, he went to synagogue during the High Holidays, and maintained traditional Jewish rituals. But I didn't know if he had any actual belief in the mystical force behind these customs. And, knowing how limited time was, I felt no need to hold back.

At first, his answer was as indirect as expected. But with tear-glazed eyes, my father told me what he felt.

✴

The three siblings stood in the synagogue, facing the *bema* — the raised platform for the Torah. Side by side, they traced their fingers along the Hebrew lines of *Mi Sheberach*, the Jewish prayer for the sick. "Oh God, who blessed our ancestors ... send your blessings to all who are ill. Have mercy on them and graciously restore their health and strength."

The Toronto synagogue was packed with the typical congregation. Soft lights illuminated the upholstered benches. Daylight filtered through stained glass. It was a Saturday morning, February 15, 1975. There might have been a bar mitzvah that day, a boy reading the Torah for the first time, although Harvey and his siblings wouldn't remember for sure.

Some couples spoke in hushed whispers, prayer books covering their faces, their chatter barely audible beneath the droning Hebrew of the rabbi who arched before a podium. Harvey stood with his tallis, a white shawl stitched with Hebrew lettering, cloaked around him. He flipped through the pages of his prayer book next to his brother and sister.

I'm not sure what he was thinking at this point. Maybe, standing in this holy sanctuary, he wondered what type of God would take two parents away from three innocent kids.

Max had never returned home after being admitted for his recent round of chemo that week. The previous night, Louise, Earl, Harvey, and Louise's husband, Howie, had visited him in the hospital.

Max was in a semi-comatose state. Howie, accustomed to seeing patients die, had told the siblings that he wouldn't be leaving that bed. But they didn't know how near death he was. Desperation had brought them to this sanctuary of prayer.

Eventually, one of the congregants, a friend of Max, whispered for the three siblings to follow him outside. The rabbi joined them in the lobby. Someone had called the shul and shared the news. Their father had just passed.

❖

Lying down on the hallway floor next to Dad's room, waiting to assist him on his next trip to the bathroom, I pulled out my phone, opened the Google Docs app, and began to write in the journal document I'd been filling since his diagnosis.

"When someone hears the dreaded, three-letter G-word, they may feel a pang of belief or disbelief," I wrote. "They may see what they must prove or disprove. They may see a debate, an argument, or some sort of Santa Claus in the clouds, puppeteering the antics of the world below, arbitrarily choosing the recipients of misery and fortune. They may list a ledger of all the ways they've been wronged in their life, all the moments of suffering and pain that seemingly disqualify the validity of a Master of the Universe protecting them. Or they may list all the things they're grateful for, and all the harmonious reasons that sanctify their spiritual convictions. I'm no preacher, and I have no interest in weighing in now."

"Do you believe in God?" I had asked my father, moments before I began writing on the hallway floor.

"All the love I've received," he replied, lifting his head to look at me in the darkness. "The family I have … It makes it hard not to."

Maybe love is, and always has been, all the proof we need.

Peanut Butter
June 8, 2020

Around three in the morning, I went to check on Dad after his visit to the bathroom. After I tucked him in, and before I flicked off the light, I noticed his eyes examining the photos on the wall in front of him. "We've got to get one of you and me," he said. There were plenty of family photos with both of us in them, but none with just the two of us.

"I'll be right back." I went downstairs to the living room and retrieved the framed photo of my dad and me sitting in a canoe from September 2017. I propped it in front of the TV.

"You're a genius," my father rasped. We held hands for a long time as we gazed at the photo. He looked at it intently. And the other photos, too. It almost felt like he was reminding himself what he was fighting for. I didn't want to let go of his hand. I didn't want him to let go of mine. We lingered there for a moment longer than normal, and I remembered that day we drifted in that canoe.

Rocking gently, I spread a glob of peanut butter with a plastic knife on a slice of white bread. The canoe drifted over small waves, and birds sang amidst the buzzing of cicadas. A light breeze swayed the tips of the tallest trees. The day was young. The sky was clear. It was two and a half years before his diagnosis, and life was as simple as a father and son eating peanut butter sandwiches on a lake.

"Roman kings never ate this well," Dad said, sitting backward at the bow's seat so his body was facing me. He held up his half-eaten sandwich close to his Oakley sunglasses on his face, like he was assessing a bar of gold in the sunlight. "What we've got here is the equivalent of caviar and champagne."

"Why certainly, good sir," I said, in a pathetic attempt at a British accent. "Did you tell the butlers to prepare our yacht for departure?"

"They have been notified, good sir," he said, in a slightly more pathetic attempt — it sounded more like an Indian accent.

I twisted the lid shut on the Kraft peanut butter jar. Then I grabbed hold of my paddle, catching it before it slid off the gunwales, gripping my sandwich in the other hand. Dad chomped into his, barely chewing before each swallow.

For a moment, as our boat rocked over waves and crumbs sprinkled onto the canoe's wet floor, I noted how much older he'd begun to look recently. Speckles of grey had appeared amidst his mostly black, receding hair. His wrinkles had sunk deeper into his tanned skin; the lines on his forehead were more pronounced. He was sixty-five then. Still, there was a youthfulness to him, a child-like vigour, that became more apparent as he delighted in the nostalgic simplicity of a peanut butter sandwich.

Such appreciation was perfectly in character; he displayed similar enthusiasm for a plate of mac and cheese, a heated frozen pizza, or a microwaved TV dinner. (Even a bowl of Corn Flakes and skim milk had him verbally thanking God.) But something about this sandwich, on this warm summer day, warranted a different type of gratitude. Maybe it was because the two slices of white bread and Kraft peanut butter offered a comforting reminder of the grass-stained days of his childhood, those adolescent summers of bike rides and track and field when caviar and champagne were foreign concepts. (Not that they would become typical indulgences later on.) Or maybe it was because, with organic alternatives dismissed, a peanut butter sandwich was one of the few things in life that remained the same.

The day prior, we had visited Mattawa and walked into the movie theatre his parents had built. One of the employees had asked us if we'd like to see the projector room, but Dad couldn't get out of there fast enough. He seemed to be haunted by how different it all felt. We headed back to the motel that night, went to sleep, and rose early the next morning to come here: Champlain Provincial Park, twenty minutes outside of Mattawa, right near the road where Dad was hit by a car when he was eleven years old.

We drifted for hours, feeling like time had slowed down. We asked some strangers — a father and son fishing — to take a picture of us, wanting to capture the moment.

As I looked at that framed photo, with its glass reflecting my frail father lying on his bed, I still tasted the sweet peanut butter on my tongue and felt the hot sun on my face. I was beguiled by that illusive spell of finding forever in a moment that would expire. As I write these words now, I feel my father's hand grasping mine. I wonder how many of the moments we look back on are moments that, while being lived, had us looking back as well. How many memories do we have of recalling memories?

I think it's okay to close our eyes and remember, so long as we open them again to see what's immediately before us.

Hockey
June 9, 2020

After spending the day with Earl, Dad showed his brother his watch collection. Too many watches collected dust in his dresser drawers — most of them cheap knockoffs. He had collected them over the decades, appreciating each purchase for the material of the strap, or the detailing of the face, or the inner mechanics. He had a passion for the watches' artistry, the way the rugged accessories depicted varying shades of masculinity. Some of his watches, unreflective of my father's relatively tame lifestyle, were crafted to withstand tough conditions, like those experienced by a deep-sea diver, or a triathlete — these were waterproof and compass-equipped. Others, with Roman numerals and more sophisticated designs, conveyed the sleek elegance of James Bond.

Lying on his bed, with Earl sitting on a chair and me fetching watch after watch, he gave each one a rambling introduction, like he was presenting an artifact in a museum.

"Now, just remember ... they don't sell this one anymore ... this one's a special edition," he said, showing one of his favourites: a watch with a sun and moon emblem on the face, atop the exposed inner mechanics. He shone a cellphone light over it to illuminate the more intricate detailing.

"And you found it at Winners," Steph called.

"Yup."

"And it's real?" Uncle Earl asked.

"Real enough," Dad replied with a shrug and smile.

Uncle Earl chuckled.

Dad's arm muscles had completely atrophied, now just sagging flesh on bones, and his skin had taken on a greyish tone, contrasting starkly with the neon T-shirt he wore. His voice was a little more hoarse and strained. Despite all this, he was exceedingly good at making those around him forget the bleakness of the situation.

A few weeks before, he and Uncle Earl had watched a vintage replay of the 1987 Canada Cup hockey game, Canada versus the Soviet Union, with Wayne Gretzky and Mario Lemieux. Keeping their distance from each other, they cheered and shouted with every goal, engrossed in the action as if it were happening in real time.

"*Here's Lemieux poking at the centre!*" yelled the commentator over the swelling applause of the arena's crowd. "*Lemieux ahead to Gretzky! There's Gretzky with another two on one ... To Lemieux ... He shoots ... He scores!*"

Harvey and Earl jolted into applause as the stadium erupted.

"*Mario Lemieux! With one-twenty-six remaining!*"

Streamers flew. Horns blasted. Signs were hoisted and fans screamed.

The commentator reiterated the action during the replay. *"This was a three-on-one break! Murphy the Wheelman ... Murphy, Gretzky, back to Lemieux — he's allowed to get right in close and pick the corner on the glove side! The glove side, high! You don't give Lemieux that kind of room!"*

"What a play!" Dad called on his bed, smiling.

"One-twenty-six remaining!" Earl called, sitting on the chair next to him.

Hockey had always been part of the two brothers' lives. There was that backyard rink their father had built in Mattawa, those Saturday mornings of blades scraping ice, snowflakes billowing around them as they reached for a gliding puck.

There were the games they watched together, both the professional ones that were televised and the much less athletic ones played by family members (such as myself), where they'd remain side by side, rooting for whichever team, sitting on bleachers or couches, applauding every goal or save. (With professional games, Dad had a tendency to start cheering for whatever side was winning in the third period, abandoning any original allegiance.)

There were also the games we all watched together. After Passover Seders at our house every year, before dessert, every guy in my family — and Steph — would report to the living room to watch the Leafs battle it out (most of the time unsuccessfully). Uncles, cousins, and fathers, all of us bloated from a three-course meal, would gather on couches and the pillowed floor, eyes glued to the buzzing TV.

Dad would often doze off shortly after the first period, then snap awake for a breakaway. "Ya, just throw it away!" he'd call, frustrated by a missed opportunity. "Wide open net, and you just bang it against the boards! Let's go, Habs! Let's go, Habs!"

"How about some loyalty, Dad?" I'd call with a smile.

"Those assholes don't deserve loyalty!"

"Tied game now!" someone would call.

"Go, Leafs, go!" Dad would shout.

The love of the game has long been a source of bonding for my family. Three periods of play. Two benches of players. Hope for a win. Fear of a loss. And a ticking clock reminding everyone time is running out.

Thank You
June 10, 2020

"I don't often say it ... or I don't often adequately say it ... but I can tell you that everything I have ... which is so amazing ... is from you," Dad told his sister, with tears building in his yellowed eyes.

Dad wanted his sister to know how much she meant to him, how much her efforts to keep the family intact those years after they lost their parents had made him who he was. Over the years, Aunt Louise had made weekly efforts to host her brothers for Friday-night dinners and made sure to include them in every birthday celebration, family gathering, and holiday. The little girl who once obsessed over fallout shelters had spent a lifetime keeping her loved ones close.

Seeing her start a family with Howie is what made Harvey want a family of his own. His love of being an uncle for three rambunctious boys grew into a desire to become a father. With his voice weaker than ever, Harvey expressed his gratitude as he lay on the living-room couch, his family gathered around him. He looked into his big sister's eyes and took her hands.

"I want you to know that I acknowledge your role. It's not often that a sister keeps a family together like that. At that age. You kept us together. Thank you from the bottom of my heart. Whatever I have, I want to thank you."

After sobbing loudly, Louise regained her composure. "We're going to be bugging you now in the mornings, too," she told her brother.

"There's an open shift at two thirty," Dad said, smiling. "It's only open from two thirty to three." Dad looked at me. "Mitchell will appreciate the time off."

❋

On a Friday night in October 1986, Harvey took Arlene's hand and knocked on the door of his sister's home. It opened, and Louise stood before them with open arms.

Years had passed since Harvey and his siblings had buried their father. He was now a personal injury lawyer, with a passion for helping people. He was proud to introduce his siblings to the women he had fallen in love with.

At Louise's home, her three children ran around. Harvey adored his nephews. (Daniel was three, Matt was seven, and Sandon was eleven.) Eventually, sitting around a table, Louise, Howie, Earl, Harvey, and Arlene toasted their glasses of wine to new beginnings.

The seeds of a new family tree were planted that day. When most young men or women fall in love, a major milestone is introducing their partner to their parents — or at least one of them. Harvey didn't have that luxury, but he was thankful, and lucky, for the family he still had.

Floss
June 10, 2020

Dad sat on a stool in the bathroom and struggled to floss. It was difficult for him to even break the thread, but he kept trying with stubborn perseverance. It was about more than dental hygiene for him. After already needing his son to help him put on his adult diapers, he was clinging onto his last bit of independence.

"Dad, it's okay to allow me to help," I offered softly.

He broke the thread and proceeded.

Shortly after his father died, Dad went to dental school in Toronto, and something happened which would haunt him for the rest of his life. In first year, he failed a final examination, which required him to retake the entire, year-long course. It was a gold inlay practical exam, a test he had felt sufficiently prepared for. Learning he failed devastated him, but learning that the five other Jewish students in his cohort also failed that same exam made him feel like something else was going on. He found out later that his professor had tampered with his marking scheme. Dad showed evidence to the university's Governing Council — he had saved his original marks — and they permitted him to retake the year's course the following autumn. They never reprimanded the professor, though. Three of the six Jewish students took the course again. The three others, including my Dad, dropped out. (He spent decades gathering evidence for this discriminatory act but never brought it to public attention.)

After ruling out dentistry, years after losing his father, he was an orphan who felt cheated by an unforgiving world. But the support of his brother and sister pushed him forward.

A year after learning he had failed, when he was still technically enrolled in the dentistry program, he wrote the LSAT and was admitted to the law school at the University of Western Ontario in London, Ontario. After graduating, he decided to pursue personal injury law, advocating for those in road accidents or life-threatening circumstances that were the result of public negligence. Eventually, he started his own practice in Toronto.

Dad's life had been full of tremendous challenges. But his adversity had never defined him. He never played the role of a victim. He never dwelled in despair or complained about how unfair his life was. He kept his head up, eyes forward, and heart open. He never took life too seriously, and he tried to make people smile or laugh every chance he got — sometimes doing so at his own expense. He kept loved ones close, and he always strived to do his best. ("All you can do is your best," he'd always tell my sister and me.) His resilience has stuck with him to this moment, as he struggled to pull a thread between his teeth.

After he rinsed his mouth, I helped Dad to bed.

Stubble on My Face
June 11, 2020

"How do you stay strong?" Mom asked Dad one night.

Through the crack of the door, I watched her kneel next to his bed, shadowed in darkness.

"I just remember what we started," Dad said. "And I remember what will continue after us."

❉

That night, I shaved my beard because I wanted Dad to see my face again before he died. I also wanted him to see how I felt — as afraid and vulnerable as a child. After tucking him in, I said good night and added, as I always did, "Tomorrow will be a good day."

"It will…. And you know what, Mitch?"

"What?" I said, bracing for a dad joke.

"It will be good after I die, too."

After he said this, I kneeled next to his bed, and his hand brushed my back, comforting me like I was a little kid.

I told him he'd see his mother again. I didn't know if I believed in heaven, but I needed him to. I wanted that conviction to ease him as his body slowly failed him. I wanted it to make the approaching endgame a little less daunting.

He had always talked about how he lived on through us. I needed to believe it more than just symbolically, more than just a phrase. I needed to believe that the compassion, the devotion, the love, would truly live on.

And maybe it would. Maybe the memory of his fatherly imprint was as promising, as enduring, as an afterlife. I knew there was something about how loved he made me feel that truly doesn't just perish. I saw it in how I cared for him now, how I carefully adjusted his pillows, how I sat with him when I knew he was scared, how I held his hand and whispered that I love him.

His compassion was already running through me. The goodness of who he was is the goodness of who I am. With the stubble on my face growing quickly, I knew my father's afterlife was the life that I would continue to live.

The Last Step
June 12, 2020

We had ordered a hospital bed for the house, but it was slow to arrive. More and more, Dad was losing his mobility and needed help getting off the toilet and getting back on. I had begun changing his diapers with swift efficiency, and Dad would tell me I was "a pro."

Mom, Steph, and I had taken turns feeding him, washing him, clothing him, and simply being next to him. Daniel, Earl, Howie, and Norman, the doctors of the family, rarely left the house. They had taken the last two weeks off from their shifts, knowing that Dad wouldn't have much more time than that. The palliative team had adjusted his pain management medication and changed his consumption time based on his pain level charts Mom had been diligently maintaining.

Today, Dad walked upstairs for the last time. He struggled to climb each step as Mom, Steph, and I cheered him on. I stayed closely behind him. His back was bonier than ever. He had lost almost all of his upper body muscle. His legs were swollen, his calves struggled to activate. He shimmied upward, grasping the banister.

"Don't stop, Dad!" Steph called. "Don't stop now!"

"There's like a million steps!" Dad groaned.

"Keep going!" I called.

"C'mon, Harvey! You can do this!" shouted Mom.

"Don't stop now! Don't stop! You can't stop now!"

As I held my arms out, ready to catch him if he fell, I remembered the night I so desperately wanted him to meet me at the top of this very staircase.

I remembered that feeling of wanting things to remain the way they once were, the desperate desire to be taken care of during a time when I was doing most of the caring.

But here was my dad, or a weakened version of him, still putting one foot in front of another as his body failed him. It made me hopeful. It made me feel that, somehow, in whatever form, in whatever circumstances, he would be waiting for me at the top of any staircase I climb.

He made it to the last step and stumbled into the upstairs bathroom.

The Proposal
June 12, 2020

Daniel and Sandon had arranged a Shabbat dinner for all of us, but Dad wasn't able to leave his bed. Their brother, Matt, had driven in from Ottawa for a final goodbye.

"Dad, Matt's downstairs," I said, hoping it would give him a burst of vitality.

"Don't believe you," Dad said.

"No, he is. Really."

"Matt's in Ottawa."

"Yeah, but he drove here to see you."

"Why would he come here?"

Emotion welled inside me. It was as if he had forgotten how little time was left, that he was dying, and his loved ones would want to say goodbye.

He couldn't summon the strength to walk, so we all gathered around him, in the room with family photos plastering the walls, and a cut-out of my article, headlined "Always Watching Over Me," pinned next to his bed.

Dad's eyes lit up when Matt walked in. "Hey, Uncle Harvey," Matt said, taking his hand.

"So good to see you," Dad said.

Besides Matt's arrival, we had another surprise for him: a personalized video message from a cast member of *Tiger King* — the zookeeper who had their arm ripped off by a tiger. It was from that website Cameo, where you pay for personal messages from B-list celebrities. My cousins had paid the hefty fee to make it happen.

Kelci Saffery sat before his webcam with a friendly smile, wearing a grey hoodie that had the words *Love Me* on the front.

"Hey, Harvey. It's Saff. And on behalf of your family, I wanted to send some positivity and personal encouragement." The zookeeper leaned closer to the webcam. "This subject, in general, touches me on a personal note because my mother did suffer with cancer, and me and my siblings lost her through it. So, I know how important it is for family to come together. And I am so honoured to be a small part of that."

Here, I found comfort in a reminder, in the well-known truth: cancer, in one way or another, has affected everyone.

Every family. Every loved one — whether it's your neighbour who lives a few houses down or a celebrity zookeeper on TV. Directly or indirectly, it has changed every life. Cancer is the antagonist we all face.

"I hope that you're keeping your head up," Saff continued. "I hope that you remember that your body is incredibly stronger than your mind gives it credit for. Just keep pushing, and always, always be your own biggest fan. Never give up on yourself."

Admittedly — and this was probably our fault for not expressing how close to the end he was — this part of the message seemed a little tone-deaf. Dad wasn't really at the point of his cancer battle where he needed a pep talk to keep fighting. A lack of motivation wasn't the problem; it was the lack of a functioning liver. But the last words Saff said made the video worth it.

"And at the end of the day, as long as you're not in a loincloth attached to a leash that's in Carole Baskin's hands, I think we're doing okay. Take care, Harvey. I wish you the best. And to your family … be strong."

Feeling a spiking pain in his rectum, Dad could only smile.

❖

After the video message, Dad read "Blessing on the Children" from his prayer book. Every Friday night, for as long as I could remember, my father read that prayer, whether we were with him or not. "This is for Stephanie," he'd say when she was on exchange in Japan. And "this is for Mitchell" he'd call when I was backpacking in South America. Distance had never lessened his devotion, and sickness wouldn't stop him now.

Struggling to trace his finger along the Hebrew lines, he spoke each word with every laborious breath. "May God bless you and keep you. May God shine light on you and be gracious to you. May God turn toward you and establish peace for you."

He was too weak to sit up to kiss my head — that was what he always did after saying the prayer when we were with him — so I kissed his head instead.

I recorded most of the evening, but I didn't record the most significant moment. It came after, once everyone was gone, when my sister and Ryan walked into the room and sat down on the edge of my father's bed.

"Dad, Ryan and I are going to be together," Steph said, her voice shaky. Mom and I overheard this down the hall and walked inside.

Dad looked up at the ceiling, alert but weak. "That will be amazing," he said. "You two are different, and that's what makes you special. I wouldn't expect Ryan to do a backflip and walk on his hands. And I wouldn't expect Steph to perform surgery. But together you form something special."

He added, "If you choose to get married, that would be great."

Steph inhaled a shuddering breath. "Dad … when we get married someday, you'll be there." She pointed to her heart. "Although we're not engaged yet … we will be someday."

Dad nodded with teary eyes.

"We will," said Ryan. "If I had a ring now ..." Then, suddenly, Ryan looked at her and said, "Steph ... will you marry me?"

They were holding hands. She was searching his eyes, to see if he meant it. He nodded. She smiled. "Yes, I will," she said, tears welling.

A surgical mask on Ryan's moustached face still remained between them, a final barrier marking the distance we had all endured in these times of hardship.

But as they stood up to leave, after Dad told the story of his proposal to Mom, Steph raised that mask off his hairy face, and kissed her new fiancé on the lips.

Index Finger
June 6, 1987

Harvey was sweating beneath his tweed jacket, fingering a small velvet box in his pants pocket. Arlene sat across from him in the dimly lit restaurant, sipping a glass of red wine, pretending not to notice her boyfriend's apparent nervousness.

The young couple were at Scaramouche, a fancy restaurant tucked in central midtown. That famous sitcom actor Al Waxman, the star of *King of Kensington*, was sitting on the level above them, attracting attention. Shortly after the plates were cleared, and shortly before dessert was served, Harvey took the velvet box out and opened it on the table, revealing his grandmother's diamond ring — a modestly sized cut, crowned on a white-gold band.

Harvey had been playing out this moment in his head for weeks prior. At one point, he considered going big with some grand romantic gesture — he even looked up prices for a hot air balloon excursion overlooking the city. He decided against it, choosing to "avoid the potential awkwardness that would come with a rejection eight-thousand feet in the air." He scaled down his plans, opting for dinner in a classy restaurant and an otherwise normal evening with the woman he had fallen in love with. It had been a year and a half since he had met Arlene at that cheese table on New Year's Eve, and he knew he wanted to build a life with her. The two small-town kids had found each other in a big city and hadn't looked back.

Her eyes watered as Harvey asked her to marry him. She nodded yes, and her tears turned to laughter when Harvey, in all his nervousness, slid the ring on the wrong finger. "Oops," he muttered, nearly knocking over a glass of wine as he pulled the ring off Arlene's index finger. She laughed.

After the mistake was corrected, Arlene held Harvey's hand over the table, feeling lighter, excited for the next chapter in a long life together.

The Familiar Soundtrack
December 2015

Years before he was sick, on a cold, winter night, with snowflakes blowing against my bedroom window, Dad knocked on my door.

"Come in," I said.

"You okay?"

I nodded.

"Move over."

I made room on my childhood bed. He lay down next to me. Hockey trophies and elementary school photos crowded my dresser. Some track and field ribbons decorated my wall next to a poster of Wayne Gretzky.

I was home from university for Christmas break, a time normally ignited with jolly spirit and the relief of a semester's end. But, on that cold, winter night, nothing jolly or relieving felt possible.

"I just … I can't believe he's gone," I said.

Dad exhaled a shuddering breath. "Your friend left this world too early."

"It feels like anyone I care about can die any second now."

He nodded, his head on a pillow. "It's normal to feel that way after something like this," he said. "All we can do is use that feeling to appreciate every moment we can. None of us will be here forever."

I sobbed. Dad kissed my head.

He gazed at the ceiling for a long time. A winter wind rolled against my window, rattling my shutters slightly.

I played a song on my phone — "To Build a Home" by Cinematic Orchestra. Playing a song that matched my sadness was the second-best therapy I knew. (The first was writing.) We listened to it as those snowflakes billowed outside, as that wind continued to roll. Dad fell asleep. He snored lightly. Then loudly. It made me smile.

I was twenty. He was sixty-one. We were two grown men lying on a childhood bed, listening to a beautiful song on a cold winter night, comforted by each other's presence, one of us so comforted that slumber took over.

Nothing more needed to be said. No words of wisdom, no fatherly lecture to ease my suffering was required. No promises about better days to come. Nothing but knowing he was with me.

His snores were a different type of song. The familiar soundtrack of being loved and protected. The music that reminded me he was by my side when the world stopped making sense.

❋

After the proposal, I opened some drawers in my parents' bedroom and looked at some of the watches. There were too many to count. He had rationalized each new purchase, saying there was a slight variation in colour of the face, or the material of the strap, or the design of the numbers or arms, or the detailing of the bezel. Whether or not such claims could be substantiated, the reality was, he simply had too many. And the irony of it all was that time was the one thing we wished we had more of.

Listening to Dad's laboured snoring through the open door, Mom, Steph, and I lay on Mom's bed. I slept between them. Steph had brought Fluffy, the stuffed doll she had when she was a little girl. In the two months that had aged us so rapidly, we were clinging onto our youth, to the comfort of our past, before it left our grip.

I listened to every snore in the room across the hall, expecting each one to be the last, expecting that familiar soundtrack of safety and protection to finally end, for the dream he'd never awake from to start.

My father's watches continued ticking in those drawers, and as we lay together, all we wanted was for them to stop.

The Brokenness of the World
June 13, 2020

In the morning, Dad and Mom called Ryan's parents to congratulate them on the engagement. Dad was weaker than ever, but miraculously, he managed to say some words. "We're so … ecstatic," he said. "After three years, I'd think there should be some progress."

Ryan's parents laughed.

"It was a beautiful moment," Steph said, after recounting the proposal.

"We should have videoed or taped it," Mom said, "but Mitchell, with his memory, wrote it down word for word."

Afterward, the family came over and we held a make-shift graduation ceremony for my master of journalism from Ryerson University (now renamed Toronto Metropolitan University). The official convocation was cancelled because of the pandemic.

My uncle Brian — Mom's younger brother — read out an email that confirmed the completion of my degree, and he handed me a rolled-up piece of blank paper. I wore my high school graduation cap for the occasion.

As Dad weakly clapped with pride, I remembered the day he learned I was admitted into the program, that day in late June of 2018 when he pointed a finger and demanded I chase my dream.

I had forgotten the password to sign into my application portal for the grad school program I had applied to six months prior, so I called the school's helpline to regain access, to check the status of my application. A woman answered. My mom was in the kitchen, so I decided I'd move to the garage. I didn't want her to overhear confirmation that I'd been rejected, that all the potential she saw in me was unfounded.

The only factor I had going for me was my portfolio — a long list of student columns and feature articles, some of which had been shortlisted for national student journalism awards. My undergraduate marks, which I failed to care about for most of my time in university, were far less impressive. I had spent more time guzzling beer than attending lectures, giving myself that archetypal advice that real education is gained from experience, not from lessons in classrooms — this would ring truer if that "experience" didn't entail puking into a frat house toilet.

"It looks like there's been an offer waiting for you since April," the woman on the helpline said.

"Offer for what?" I replied dumbly.

Just then the garage roared open. Dad's charcoal-grey Audi pulled into the driveway. The engine cut, the door swung open, and he stepped out. He wore his long black coat and was carrying a stack of legal files under one arm.

"What's up, Dad?" I called, after saying goodbye to the lady on the helpline. I was sitting on the steps leading to the laundry room door.

"About five seven," he replied, typically. "Growing horizontally," he added, also typically, patting his gut.

"Guess what … It looks like I got into that graduate program. For journalism."

He paused, registering this, and dropped the files onto the garage floor. His eyes started tearing where he stood, watering with a burst of pride I didn't expect.

"Dad … I can't accept it," I said. "I'm starting that content marketing job in three days."

It was true. I was set to become some sort of account executive for a company that built marketing campaigns with media outlets, promoting products and brands in magazines and newspapers. There had been multiple rounds of interviews, and I was lucky to get the job with no previous sales experience. Deep down, I knew this was a cop-out — I would have to set aside my journalistic ambitions in favour of the objective of corporate gain — yet, I had done some considerable mental gymnastics to convince myself that this was a good first step. The salary had sealed the deal.

Dad clenched his jaw, his eyes still tearing. He pointed a stiff finger at me. "Tell them you need to quit. They'll understand."

"Dad … I can't just …"

"Tell them you need to quit."

"I can't just quit before I even …"

"Mitch, tell them you need to quit."

Looking at me with those tearing eyes, he knew, unquestionably, what I really wanted. It was a moment of being seen, penetratingly understood, by someone who knows me best.

Dad was never one to push me to do something I didn't want to do, never one to encourage me to pursue professions in law or medicine because of the financial security those jobs afforded. He wanted me to chase my passion, to surrender to my deepest desires, to follow the love for storytelling he had seen me display throughout my lifetime — from those early fictional rambles I scribbled as a little boy, to the words I wrote to honour a lost friend.

Maybe the ultimate measure of a good parent is not just unconditional love, but a willingness to support whatever it is their children hope to become.

That pointed finger will forever be the greatest gift he gave me.

✦

Afterward, we played a video that the faculty of my program sent out to all master of journalism students. It featured instructors expressing their farewells and congratulations. At the end, one of my professors spoke about how it's the obligation of every journalist to tell stories that make people feel less alone during difficult times. Then she read out a poem by a writer named L.R. Knost. I held my mother's hand as we listened to the words, sitting on opposite sides of my dad's bed, his swollen stomach rising and falling beneath our interlocked fingers.

"Do not be dismayed by the brokenness of the world," the poem went. "All things break, and all things can be mended. So go.... The broken world waits in darkness for the light that is you."

Harvatious
June 13, 2020

While he was drifting in and out of sleep, beginning intermittent comatose, Dad was visited by his best friend, Allan. They had known each other for more than fifty years, and their friendship was kept strong by frequent calls and weekly get-togethers over coffee.

As Allan sat down on the chair next to Harvey's bed, seeing his best friend so close to the end, he exhaled slowly behind his

face mask and stayed silent for a moment. "Oh, Harvatious …
what will I do without you?" he said eventually, clasping and
unclasping his hands. "Harvatious," he said again. "I wonder
why I've always called you that."

"I know why," Mom called behind him. "*My dad* called
him Harvatious!"

And suddenly the tracing of a nickname reminded us how
connected the smallest details of someone's life can be. The
name started with my grandfather, Buddy; he'd use it out
of affection when addressing his son-in-law on the phone.
"Harvatious! How're you doing?"

Norman, Buddy's son, quickly started using the same name
as well. "Well, if it isn't Harvatious!" he'd say when greeting
him at their house for dinners.

Norman was best friends with Galla, the woman he would
introduce to Harvey's best friend, Allan, and who would become his wife. Galla, after hearing Norman, began calling
Dad "Harvatious," and soon Allan was doing it, too. "Look
out everyone! Here comes Harvatious!"

Recognizing that something as simple and ordinary as
a nickname demonstrated the lasting impact of her father
brought tears to Mom's eyes. Even after we die, she recognized,
the things we've done and the words we've used can continue
projecting into the future in little ways.

After Allan said his goodbye, I walked him to the door.
"Shitty year," he said, his face trembling with emotion. (His
mother had died the day before.) I patted him on the back and
told him I know what it's like to lose a good friend.

"It's fricken' amazing about your sister's engagement. I'm so glad he got to see that." We made it to the door. He hesitated before leaving. "I have so many memories with Harv," he said. "So many great memories."

I recalled telling Gaby's sister something similar. "I'd like to hear them sometime," I said. "I'd like to hear every story you can remember."

He nodded, and as he walked down the driveway, I realized that the weight on my shoulders — the burden to keep my father's memory alive — could be shared.

Morphine and Honey
June 13, 2020

Metal banged and clattered as I held my dad's hand and the delivery men assembled the hospital bed. The palliative team had ordered it weeks ago, but it only arrived today. We figured it was worth having if it could make Dad a little more comfortable. Knowing how terrible a condition he was in, we now realized they were assembling his deathbed.

The loud noises seemed to scare him, so I stayed by his side and played some Cat Stevens on my phone. His eyes were droopy and yellow.

After it was assembled, Daniel, Howie, Earl, and I helped transfer Dad to the new bed, carrying him by the sheets under him.

We all immediately regretted it.

He started yelling. He was uncomfortable and scared. And the new position seemed to aggravate his rectum pain more than ever. We tried to give him morphine, but he was suddenly incapable of swallowing.

Mom frantically called the Sunnybrook palliative team to see if we could get a nurse to come to the house, someone who could bring a winged infusion set (also known as a "butterfly") for hydromorphone injections.

Given the demands and protocol of the pandemic, no nurses were available on short notice, and they wouldn't be able to deliver the butterflies or the hydromorphone until the following morning.

Dad groaned in agony.

"We need them *now*!" I yelled.

"Another option is to bring him to Sunnybrook," the nurse offered. "We can give him the hydromorphone here."

At that moment, Steph, Mom, and I looked at one another and made a unanimous decision.

"He stays home," Mom said.

"He stays home," I echoed.

"He stays home," Steph said with a nod.

Mom hung up, and Daniel took the lead. In the kitchen, he and other family members began crushing up morphine pills and mixing them into plastic spoons holding globs of honey. The sweetness, Daniel figured, would cause more salivation and would therefore make the morphine easier to swallow.

Howie crushed the fifteen-milligram pills, Daniel mixed the honey, and Sandon ran the spoons to me. I tried to feed my Dad as he quivered in agony. He twitched and groaned. As I spoon-fed him the morphine, he bit my finger. My eyes watered as I tried to soothe him, my heart thudded quicker.

Louise and Earl stayed close to their brother. Stephanie squeezed his hand on the other side. Norman was on the phone trying to get access to hydromorphone in case Dad didn't absorb the honey-morphine.

For a while, it seemed like a nightmare, a final, climactic test of our nursing team's ability to care for Dad in his moment of need. Our only mission was to make him comfortable, and suddenly, when it mattered most, we were failing miserably.

But the moment of heart-thrashing chaos suddenly sputtered out, replaced by a sweet serenity. Finally, with the morphine kicking in, Dad stopped struggling and began to breathe slowly. A look of calm eased his face, and every one of us exhaled with relief.

As the minutes stretched to hours, and that calm remained, our sobs turned to conversation. I held my father's hand while each of his breaths grew shallower, and family members reminisced about the underwear-dancing, joke-telling, family-loving brother, uncle, husband, and father he was.

We talked about his compassion, how he recently settled a case on Zoom, the engagement proposal last night, the graduation ceremony that morning, how this whole nightmare brought our family closer.

And then, at exactly 7:38 p.m., Uncle Norman felt his pulse. "He's passed," he said, and a stillness filled the air.

Not Just a Body
June 13, 2020

Two men from the funeral home arrived to take away Dad's body. We said our final goodbyes in the spare bedroom upstairs. Each family member gave him a kiss.

When it was my turn, I looked into his vacant eyes and knew he was no longer there. I felt a mix of despair and appreciation. A pang of delayed disbelief mingled with a sense of gratitude. I was thankful that all his suffering was over.

"I love you more," I whispered in his ear before kissing his head. "And don't argue."

Shortly after, the two men came in and covered his face with a body bag. Before they loaded him in the van, I asked one of them to read the article I wrote in the *Globe*. I wanted them to have some idea of who they were taking away.

One of the guys sat at the bench at the front door and read the column. His eyes softened with emotion as the paper crinkled in his hands.

After he finished, I told him that I don't want my father to be "just another body." Just another delivery load to transport to the funeral home.

He stood and looked directly into my eyes, bearing a sympathetic expression that matched Dr. Petrella's on that day she told Dad and me there was nothing we could do. "Let me tell you something," he said. "I've been doing this for years. And it's *never* just another body. I remember every mother and father I've taken away. I just can't forget them."

Here was a man whose vocation was dealing with death, working during a time in history when his service was in particularly high demand. He was someone who carried much more than the weight of dead bodies, and as he reassured me how much he cared, I knew Dad was in good hands.

After they loaded him into the truck and closed the back doors, I stood alone next to the front lawn and watched the tires reverse onto the road with a crunch on pavement. Then, for the last time, Dad drove away from home.

Funeral
June 15, 2020

It was a blue-sky day, and the funeral director granted us a little extra time for the graveside service, despite tight pandemic restrictions enforcing twenty-minute time slots. Steph spoke first, then Mom, then me. Louise and Earl shared some words after.

Crowd size was also limited, so I was only able to invite some of my best friends. Coby, Sam, and Mike stood together. Next to them was a short girl with eyes that resembled someone I missed dearly.

I had invited Sabrina to the funeral after she sent me a story the night my father died. It was about her and Gaby as little kids and was her way of saying she would be there for me the way I was for her. Unlike everyone else who was wearing formal black attire, Sabrina wore a baggy hoodie with fraternity letters on the front. It was as if to remind me that her brother was also mine. Today, as that brother welcomed my father, his sunlight was shining down on us.

After the casket was lowered into the grave, Mom, Steph, and I lifted a shovel from the mound of dirt. Two at a time, family members grabbed shovels. Dirt sprinkled onto the tanned wood of the coffin with loud thuds. The funeral director told us time was almost up, but the job wasn't done. Norman grabbed the shovel. Then came Howie. Then Louise and Earl. Friends helped after; the pile of dirt slowly rose.

Eventually, with the hole mostly filled, we were told that the cemetery employees would do the rest. During a time when everything had slowed down, we walked to our cars, reminded of how much it sucked to be rushed.

Transmission Speech
June 15, 2020

After the burial, we held a shiva on Zoom at the house for everyone who couldn't come to the limited-sized funeral. After prayers, friends and family were unmuted to share memories of Harvey. Allan told a couple of funny stories about Dad, and he initiated some healthy laughter.

Eventually, I played one of the audio recordings from the many interview sessions I conducted, and Dad was able to give everyone some final words after he was buried.

"I tried to give my family the best I could," he said. "But I've gotten back, in terms of pride, and love, more than I gave you. And if there is any interruption in that, if something happens to me, you have to understand … that transmission will continue."

The screen was a grid of muted, crying faces framed in little squares.

"You and Steph will have children. And the love I gave you will be transmitted to them. And you'll get back what I have gotten. No one can live forever, but I want to. I want to be there for you *forever*." The audio captured a sniffle and a long exhale. "I want to enjoy the things that you enjoy. I want to enjoy children, and grandchildren, and your accomplishments. And I'm hoping I will be able to. But if anything happens where I'm not, you must understand … you saw the transmission between me and you…. What about the transmission between me and my parents?

"The love that they gave me stayed with me long after they died. The love I give you will stay with you, too. Because that love is immortal. That love will bring us together no matter what's happening in the world. No matter the circumstances that keep us apart."

I remembered the night Gaby died, when I wrote his obituary. I remembered thinking that words are what anchor our existence to the ground and prevent us from drifting away. As I listened to my father's recording, seeing all the teary eyes on the little squares of the computer screen, I realized it's not the words that secure our existence to the ground but the love that writes them down.

The Tears of Night
April 2017

The professor stood at the front of the lecture room and began to weep softly.

It was my last class of my undergraduate degree, a literary theory course that required us to carry around a book too big to fit in any normal backpack, the second edition of *The Norton Anthology of Theory and Criticism*. It was loaded with fancy terms like "formalism" and "structuralism" and "postmodernism." It was, unsurprisingly, a dry course. But Dr. Poetzsch made it better.

He was a tall man, in his forties, I think, with spiked blond hair and hipster glasses. There was a warmth in his eyes, and he imparted a graceful eloquence to every lecture. His love for literature was contagious.

During the last class of the year, as spring sunshine beamed through a dusty window, he read us a passage from Nobel laureate Elie Wiesel's *Night*. It was from a scene toward the end of the book, when Elie, a sixteen-year-old Jewish prisoner of wartime concentration camps that included Auschwitz and Buchenwald, said a final goodbye to his father — in the barracks of a camp crowded with corpses. His father's will to live was drained; he was broken, exhausted, and sick. Elie had given him his rations of soup, desperate to keep him alive. But his father would not go on. Familiar with what the surrender to death appeared like, Elie etched every detail of his father's battered face in his memory before leaving him to die.

As powerful as the passage was, it was the way in which Dr. Poetzsch read it that struck me so deeply. His chest shuddered. His eyes watered. He struggled to keep reading; each word was broken by soft sobs. He continued despite this, enunciating every stomach-punching word. The class of senior students, young men and women in our early twenties, watched this with amazement. This wasn't a performance. It wasn't his first time reading the passage. But Dr. Poetzsch was genuinely moved to tears.

The moment is hard to forget. It inspired me to look at literature and the pursuit of writing in an entirely new way. Writing, I understood from then on, was not only a medium for lyricism, or wit, or persuasiveness, it offered a means for real, profound communication between a writer and a reader, one that could transcend the borders academia and criticism tried to create for it, one that could reach far beyond the labels of "formalism," "structuralism," "postmodernism," and all the other terms literary theorists like to use. Literature, I realized, was a form of telepathy, a connective dialogue that somehow communicated something beyond language, something strong enough to expose the darkest of nights, something poignant enough to make a grown man cry in front of a room of students, cutting through the armour that shields vulnerability, and making the loss of someone's father feel like the loss of your own.

❋

I thought about that moment with Dr. Poetzsch the night after the funeral, as I lay awake, habitually waiting to hear the groan of the floorboard outside Dad's room, knowing full well that I wouldn't. In an attempt to calm my turbulent mind, I grabbed my phone, which rested on a tall stack of books on my night table, and, yet again, began to write.

"I think stories are about permission," I typed. "Permission to feel what you want — or need — to feel. Permission to explore your grief, to acknowledge your trauma, to discover your joy. To ascend beyond your immediate experience and find yourself floating before someone else's. I think the best stories give you permission to be both who you are and someone else. They permit you to find new worlds, merge paths with lost souls, and climb the most desolate towers. They are a calling chant for adventure, a shout on a rollercoaster, a spiritual unloading of what dwells deep inside us and causes us to tremble with hope and jump with ecstasy and floor the gas pedal as we scream out our rage. Stories are the permission we yearn for to find new roads no matter where we're seated, no matter the circumstances that lock us indoors. They launch us forward, turn us around, and bound us off the tarmac onto bumpy and often unpredictable terrain. They can make us dance in our underwear, smile in the face of despair, tell silly jokes, cry when all hope is lost. And they carry us into the darkness, revealing the tears of night while casting the sunshine of better days."

The words of L.R. Knost rattled through my mind that night: "The broken world waits in darkness for the light that is you."

The light is you, Dad, I thought. The light is you.

Purpose
July 23, 1992

The white fluorescent lighting of a hospital room illuminated Arlene as she lay on the bed, tense from contractions. "Harv," she said, her brown hair a mess over her sweaty face. "Tell me that story to make me laugh."

"Which one?"

"The one about the garbage bags … the sexy legs contest."

Harvey, who was holding her hand, leaned closer and told the story as a few nurses prepared Arlene for delivery. He placed one hand on her rounded stomach, protruding beneath the hospital gown.

"Okay … here it goes. There was a big company party at that insurance firm I was working at. Wellington Insurance. It was '86. Or was it '87?" Harvey started counting backward in his head, pointing to his fingers.

"Doesn't matter, Harv," Arlene said after a long moment.

"No … no … it was '86."

"Completely irrelevant, Harvey!"

"Yeah, yeah. Eighty-six. Maybe '87. Don't know. Anyway, at one point, one of the senior managers thought it would be funny for a bunch of the male staff to stand on the stage with garbage bags over their heads. They must've cut out holes in them, so they could breathe. The idea was for the crowd to guess whose legs were whose, and to cheer for whoever had the sexiest legs. So, one by one, the applause got louder or quieter, depending on the contestant who stepped forward with rolled-up pants and a garbage bag covering their upper-half. And guess who got the the loudest applause? 'Harvey wins!' they shouted. 'Consky's got the sexiest legs!' The whole place went *nuts*. They cheered and applauded. But when they removed the garbage bag, it wasn't even me. Could've been the mailman. The intern, for hell's sake. Because I wasn't even there."

"Where were you?" Arlene asked, giggling, already knowing the answer.

"There was a sale at The Bay."

She laughed.

Then she squeezed his hand. "I'm scared, Harv," she said.

"You'll do great," Harvey said, before kissing her stomach.

Moments later, Arlene was rolled into the delivery room. And at exactly eight twenty-five on Wednesday morning, a baby girl was born. She weighed six pounds, nine ounces, but felt much lighter as she wailed in Harvey's arms for the first time.

Sunlight filtered through an open window, and Harvey watched the infant adjust to the recovery room's light with half-closed eyes. He couldn't believe something so small would grow into a real human. As Harvey rocked her gently, the wailing stopped, and the baby named after his mother wrapped her little hand around his thumb.

It was then that something changed in him. He felt a buoyancy, a lightness that filled his chest and relaxed his shoulders. It was a feeling unlike anything he had ever experienced, like a breeze of serenity filling each breath. It was as if holding this small bundle of flesh and bones, an extension of himself, and an extension of his own parents, was like holding the secret to pure happiness.

"It just had a magical, magical sense to it," he would recall twenty-eight years later, with an iPhone capturing every word resting on a nightstand crowded with pill containers and family photos plastering surrounding walls. "We had created this beautiful being … It was the strangest thing … The *strangest* thing."

He felt that this singular moment made any pain, any suffering from the past or future, entirely worth enduring. A sense of deep purpose settled the moment Harvey became Dad.

The Projector Screen
August 19, 2020

Two months after my father passed, our family walked into the old movie theatre in Mattawa.

It was pretty much the same as when Dad and I had visited a few years prior. The time-machine mosaic of film memorabilia included movie posters dating back to the seventies and eighties. That dusty glass cabinet loaded with film reels rested next to the rusted projector, in a shadowed display section that now looked more like a forgotten storage unit. I glanced at the *Rocky II* poster I had noticed years before, with a beaten Sylvester Stallone struggling to stay upright in a boxing stance and imagined my father giving me his best Rocky impersonation: "It ain't about how hard you hit. It's about how hard you can get hit and keep moving forward."

Wearing masks, Louise and Earl wandered around the place they spent much of their youth. It was their first time back in decades. "The snack bar was on the other side," Earl recalled. "And that washroom used to be the ticket office."

I had contacted the current owner of the theatre a couple weeks prior, when we first decided to take the road trip to Mattawa. She agreed to open the doors for us, despite the theatre being closed during the pandemic. The manager, Lyse, met us at the front door a little before sundown. As she showed us around, Earl and Louise asked her the same question my father did years ago: "Do you guys use Savoral on the popcorn kernels?"

"We use Flavacol!" Lyse said. "It's the same stuff. The company changed the name a bunch of years ago."

I smiled, knowing my father would find relief in the preservation of that minor detail.

Lyse opened up the door at the end of the foyer, and we walked into a dark auditorium with its four hundred and twenty-two faded-cherry seats. The screen was the same screen, Lyse told us, that Max and Sandra installed when they first built the theatre.

Matt's son Benjamin ran jubilantly down the aisles, and Daniel and Matt chased him. As they did, Lyse told Earl and Louise how important the theatre was to their community. She said she remembered first seeing *Jaws* here in 1975. "I wouldn't get in the water for the rest of that summer."

I asked if I could see the projector room. She checked her pockets. "Unfortunately, I don't have the keys."

I told myself I'd need to come here another time.

Eventually, the family filed out, but I lingered alone in the darkened auditorium, brushing my hand over the cherry-coloured seats. I looked at the screen, the same one my father watched all those movies on growing up, and felt a sense of satisfaction, knowing that my quest to learn about his past was far from over and recognizing that some things — popcorn seasoning, a projector screen, an old movie theatre — can withstand the tidal wave of time, memorializing the people and memories we fear will become too pixelated to recall and serving as tangible reminders of a presence that still endures. My favourite line from *Tuesdays with Morrie* came to mind: "Death ends life; not relationships."

Afterward, the family got into our three cars and drove to the cabin we were staying in, twenty minutes outside of town. We accelerated north, down the old Highway 543. The Mattawa River glimmered with moonlight to the right, seen through the August leaves that shadowed both sides of the road. Uncle Earl, who was sitting in the passenger seat of the car I was in, told me his family would drive down this road on summer nights and head to their old cottage. I imagined my father sitting between his two siblings, with his parents at the front, moving along the same road, their high beams cutting through darkness.

When we got back to the cabin, we stoked the wood furnace and retired on a cluster of musty couches. Matthew carried Benjamin to bed and read him a story before joining us. With the fire crackling, Daniel asked his mom why she never spoke about her parents.

"I guess it just caused me too much pain," Louise said. "There's a lot of conversations I wish we could've had when Harvey was here."

"We can have them now," Earl said.

Eventually, after a couple hours of Louise and Earl sharing memories of their past, we all went upstairs to a small room where all the beds were. It was a close space, with thick walls and dusty air. Daniel was convinced the cabin was an Ayahuasca retreat centre. I thought it looked like a fallout shelter.

My eyelids grew heavy, and with the breathing of my family rising and falling around me, their light snores filling the close space, I drifted off to sleep, feeling what I hoped my father felt during his final days. Safe.

Epilogue: Father's Day
June 19, 2022

Standing before a mirror in a vineyard villa, I struggled to thread my tie into a double Windsor knot.

"Take the longer end on the left, and, with your left hand, bring it back over the triangle and through the loop," said the man in the YouTube tutorial video, to my complete frustration.

With my phone propped up on the sink counter, I had been following steps one to five, but the sixth and seventh steps were only tying my brain in a knot. My navy-blue tie was a tangled mess.

A single Windsor was something I could normally pull off, but I'd accidentally brought a white dress shirt with a wider collar split, and that required a thicker knot. Dad would've been the guy to fix this.

For every special occasion that required a tie, he was always there to straighten it out, to tighten away the wrinkles, and to get the length just right.

He pulled it straight the night of my prom, something for which I was grateful even if it inevitably loosened after I guzzled too much Captain Morgan. He centred it the day of my high school graduation before I walked on stage and was awarded my diploma. He smoothed out the seams for my undergraduate convocation and adjusted the length of the tail when I prepared for my first job interview.

But now all I had was Ben from the *My Nice Tie* tutorials.

Well, that's not really true.

Once I realized the collar mistake, I made a couple of calls. First I dialed Uncle Earl, who was driving to the venue and didn't pick up. Then I called my older cousin Sandon, who was in the car with Uncle Howie. They struggled to instruct me through grainy FaceTime reception but ultimately resorted to sending a few YouTube videos for me to try alone.

After I pulled something together that was a little less disastrous than prior attempts, I splashed some water on my face and walked to the entrance of the vineyard.

Uncle Howie, who had just arrived, found me quickly — and he undid my mangled attempt, weaving the tie into a thick double Windsor to spare me further embarrassment.

The experience offered a reminder: there is more than one elder in a lifetime to guide you through its many confusions. It was a fitting lesson for that particular day.

Steph and Ryan were getting married on Father's Day.

They didn't plan it deliberately. It just sort of fell into place. They had chosen to wait two years for pandemic restrictions to subside, and Father's Day Sunday was the only availability at the venue. We decided it would be a way to honour him, turning a day that would be otherwise dominated by his absence into one of celebration and joy.

They had discovered a winery about a forty-minute drive northeast of Toronto, and chose to seal the deal amidst vineyard villas, between two weeping willow trees that crowned a rippling pond.

Four posts of cedar wood, squared by four beams at the top, would serve as the *chuppah*, a raw-bone structure that, in Jewish tradition, symbolizes the first home of the newlyweds. I had assembled it early that morning, drilling four-inch screws into the cedar wood to connect the pieces. I'd also hung a canopy of white fabric on the top, and beneath it, strung my father's tallis to flap gently in the spring breeze. (And I could hardly tie a tie.)

Shortly after guests arrived, following a burst of captured photos, sunlight poked through scattered clouds as I walked my only living grandparent down the grassy aisle. Uncle Earl held Bubbie's left arm and I held her right as she smiled gracefully at the rows of guests sitting on white chairs.

After making it to the end, I took my place beneath my dad's tallis, standing across from Ryan, his parents, and two sisters, inside the *chuppah* that overlooked the pond. A soft breeze rolled in. Then, a heavier wind. The four wooden posts of the *chuppah* shook slightly. As the fabric canopy began to whip like the sails of a boat, I was suddenly horrified that the structure that symbolized the first home of Steph and Ryan, the one that I had constructed, would fall.

The day was not without some laughable fumbles. Before Ryan walked down the aisle, the music wouldn't play on the speakers. The cantor, who was officiating the wedding, whipped out a guitar to kill the awkward silence, but his music sheets kept flying away. In a distant parking lot, someone's car beeped a minute too long. A few loose tissues littered the aisle, distorting the florist's carefully manicured aesthetic. And now, the *chuppah* was threatening to collapse. And the brother of the bride would be to blame.

C'mon Dad, I thought. *Help me out here.*

I've talked to him often throughout the last two years — sometimes during long walks, sometimes during long car rides. The many audio recordings I saved served as suitable relief for those moments I needed to actually hear a reply.

I wish I could say that losing my father was the only tragedy that struck my family throughout the dark days of the pandemic. But the truth was there was another vacancy at my sister's wedding, another loss that shook our home.

Eight months after my dad's passing, Uncle Norman died of a heart attack. I had seen him hours before it happened, while lifting weights in his basement with his son, my younger cousin, Maor — who, choosing to follow his father's footsteps, had been accepted to medical school a week prior.

Uncle Norman's abrupt end offered a jarring juxtaposition to my father's passing. Although the speed of my dad's decline was capable of giving us whiplash, we were blessed with final moments and the closure that arrives with anticipation. Norman didn't get to say goodbye.

Those cedar posts were rocking a little more as my mother, who lost her husband and brother within eight months, walked to the halfway point of the aisle, wearing a navy-blue dress that matched my suit and tie and beaming a joyful smile that did not match the pain she'd endured over the last two years. Like she did every day since losing two great men, she put one foot in front of the other, and her smiling eyes welcomed the loved ones who surrounded her. Then, as my mother stopped walking, the music changed.

The song that played was an instrumental arrangement for piano by musician Max Arnald, a cover of the song "I'm Yours," originally by Jason Mraz. The melancholic but hopeful melody ascended as seated guests turned towards the vineyards behind them.

And that's when Stephanie stepped forward. Her face glowed with that infectious smile she'd had since we were little kids. Her sweeping wedding gown rippled with the breeze.

My eyes teared as Steph floated down the aisle and took Mom's hand. They walked to the *chuppah* with heads held high.

Steph's dress was purchased from The Brides' Project, an organization that sells modern wedding gowns, worn once and donated, to raise funds for cancer research. It was yet another way Steph had chosen to honour the man who should have been by her side.

As I watched her walk down the aisle, that warmth in my chest, the one I felt when my father hugged me tight or when one of his dumb jokes triggered an avalanche of laughter, expanded. The pain of loss was overpowered by something I can't really explain. It wasn't just happiness, or hope, or relief that we had reached the light at the end of a dark and winding tunnel. I'm sure the darkness won't ever be completely behind us. But a new certainty was shining through the clouds.

I glanced at my father's tallis that swung and whipped above me, and, gripping one of the cedar posts that continued to sway, I realized the simple truth behind this feeling.

With all the uncertainties of life, any home may shake. People will die. Loneliness may settle. Isolation may interfere. But something — call it love, call it a "transmission" — will keep it sturdy. Whatever this is, it could stop a home from tumbling.

And if it doesn't, it could offer the foundation to rebuild.

✤

The ceremony continued like a sweet dream. With birds chirping, the cantor read Hebrew scripture as Steph and Ryan locked eyes. The pond reflected afternoon sunlight as Ryan stomped on glass, a tradition that pays tribute to the fallen Jewish temples. Then he kissed the bride. An eruption of applause from the teary-eyed assembly followed.

The party that followed was in a large white tent with a dance floor. Shortly before the first course was served, the DJ introduced me as the MC, and I took the stage and stood before the podium microphone. Holding a glass of rum and Coke, I cracked some harmless jokes about Ryan, imparted some loving words to Steph, and then raised my glass to fathers.

"Something I have come to learn is that there is more than one father in a lifetime," I said, concluding my speech. "There are uncles, older cousins, fathers-in-law, mentors, teachers, role models. Ben from *My Nice Tie*. And there are the fathers that we will turn into. The ones who will pay the love we've received forward …

"So, on this Father's Day, I'd like us to raise our glasses to dads. To the ones we have lost, the ones we still have, and the ones we will become."

✦

Did we dance?

We danced like we were all members of the Dads Who Dance in Underwear Society. As ties were loosened (finally) and heels were abandoned, we jumped and twirled and shook along the dance floor like our bodies were possessed.

As the DJ played some Michael Jackson, I hugged Steph and Ryan tightly in the centre of the floor. Mom hugged us, too. Friends and family joined in on the embrace, kissing heads, hoisting shot glasses, basking in endless joy.

In my wedding speech, I had included a quote from one of my father's recordings, and the words repeated in my mind during that group hug.

They were words that, I believe, every son and daughter would want to hear from their old man.

"I'm just so incredibly proud," he had said.

Looking around, I knew it to be true.

Afterword
Double Milk, No Sugar

Here's the thing with photos of people you've lost. They become coloured by a melancholic tint — it's as if all those joyful moments were lies. As if the happiness of the captured memories were some sort of illusion.

If only that little boy, with cake icing covering his face, knew that, years later, he would watch his father suffer tremendously. If only that family, sitting on kayaks and paddle boards, would know how limited their time as a complete family would be. Would any of those smiles still be there? Would any of that joy remain?

This is how we look at time, through the lens of what would come. But why does the joy of our past need to be disqualified? Why does past happiness need to seem like a lie because, we come to believe later, based on our linear conceptions of existence, that future troubles negate it? Why should we feel cheated by joy?

Often, when people who are mourning walk into a familiar place, a coffee shop or restaurant they used to go with the person they lost, they feel violated. We went to this place when life was normal. We laughed and smiled and told stupid jokes. The unsuspected normality is deceptive.

We feel this way because we were doomed to lose a battle we didn't even know we were fighting. Or because it wasn't even a battle. It was an ambush. Night by night. Day by day. Or maybe the fight was lost in a few seconds. A heart attack or motorcycle accident. We feel as if the comfort and safety and security we felt in those past moments were hiding an outcome that would ultimately blindside us, concealing an end we'd remain oblivious to.

It's almost funny — I prefer remaining in the place of my father's suffering, the house where he died, to venturing to those places where he was happy and healthy. At least the house hasn't lied to me. The house warned me — with the blood on the tiled floor, the medication containers crowding table space, the faces of sorrow, the weight of fear and dread in the cool air. But the bagel shop Dad and I always used to go to early mornings, the place where we would eat cream cheese and lox before he would go off to work and I'd go to school, where he'd settle for the cheaper coffee and I'd walk a few stores down to Starbucks that was in the same plaza and return with my black medium roast, and he'd drink his instant crap with double milk and no sugar, and I'd laugh about how easily he's satisfied … that place feels like a big lie. But I know it wasn't.

I know if there's one thing the two and a half months of my father's illness taught me, it's that sadness and grief don't disqualify joy. They can accentuate it. They can make those moments feel all the more beautiful. They can alleviate the pressure to turn it all into something grand and spectacular, to calculate new horizons, to build new opportunities. In many ways, the joy feels more real now. More fragile, yes, but more miraculous, also. The past seems like a gift, one that isn't dominated by a later day.

That's all to say: moments of joy aren't a lie. They're not a grand deception that can block you from seeing what truly awaits. They are glimpses of freedom, what happens when you jump off that sequential timeline and stop looking beyond what you're seeing. Like an old movie projector flipping through film, each image leads to the next. All we could do is sit back and enjoy the show.

While you're at it, hug someone you love.

Mitch
June 2022

Acknowledgements

I have some incredible people in my life who helped this story grow from a campfire ramble to the book in your hands. Given what — and who — this memoir is about, it would be most fitting to first thank my family for allowing me to share such intimate details of their lives. My mom, Arlene Consky, and my sister, Steph Consky, offered continuous support, straining over countless re-reads of drafts, carrying out long discussions about word choices, and engaging in deep reflections on the man this book centres around, my father, Harvey Consky, who, along with my mother, is the biggest reason I call myself a writer. My new brother-in-law, Ryan Adesky, allowed me to include him in these pages and continues to be an incredible addition to our clan. My aunt Louise Shogilev and uncle Earl Consky offered substantial notes that helped sharpen the details of my dad's past, and they devoted countless hours to making this book something the family could be proud of. My uncle Howie Shogilev and cousins Daniel, Sandon, and Matt

Shogilev also offered encouragement from the beginning, and their endless love for my father pushed me to do this right. My uncle Brian Epstein read early and late drafts and has remained one of my most fierce and loyal cheerleaders, along with my grandmother (Bubbie) Eleanor Epstein, my aunt Iris Epstein, and my cousins Maor and Chantelle Epstein. My uncle Norman Epstein, who, along with my dad, this book is dedicated to, has always been a source of inspiration; the memories of his past and the absence of his physical presence encouraged me to write these words with bravery and humility.

My friends are superstars. Some of them are mentioned in these pages, others were there behind the scenes, but all of them have supported me unconditionally — whether through reading early drafts, listening to my impassioned monologues, or simply pushing me to keep writing over the years. Here's a convoluted list of them, in no particular order: Sam Milner, Michael Jacobson, Coby Samuels, Sabrina Barsky, Josh Peters, Jared Czitron, Mara Carson, Jacob Carson, Emily Sherman, Moishe Goldman, Grace Wells-Smith, Emily Latimer, Nikki Wisener, Matt Render, Jared Westreich, Ryan Nisker, Hailey Wengle, Urbi Khan, Carli Gardiner, Evan Ross, Phil Sigal, Leah Kuperman, Lena Yang, Will Huang, and Shelby Blackley.

John Parry, my first reader and editor — who I met at a coffee shop almost five years ago and who has since become one of my best friends — applied exhaustive attention to every sentence and provided unwavering encouragement since the start of the writing process. My other editor, Dominic Farrell, applied just the right touch, polishing the text to a shine and finding errors that only his trained eye would detect.

Thank you to my agent, Hilary McMahon, for taking a shot on me, and my acquisition editor, Julie Mannell, for seeing potential in my story. Laura Boyle designed the cover with great sensitivity to the story and a strong receptiveness to my input, and Erin Pinksen was a reliable line of contact throughout the whole publishing process. I'm also thankful to the rest of the Dundurn team for all the work they put into turning this word dump into an actual book.

Finally, thank you to all of the people out there who have shared their recounts of loss, grief, and resilience. Your stories are medicine for broken hearts.

About the Author

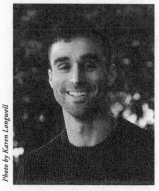

Photo by Karen Longwell

Mitchell Consky is a Toronto-based journalist with works published in the *Globe and Mail*, the *Toronto Star*, the *Walrus*, *BNN Bloomberg*, and CTV News. He specializes in long-form feature writing and essays about loss, travel, and adventure. He holds a master of journalism from Toronto Metropolitan University and a bachelor's degree in English and film from Wilfrid Laurier University. When not working, his ideal escape is drifting on a canoe in Ontario's Algonquin Park.

A portion of Mitchell's author royalties will be donated to cancer research at Sunnybrook Hospital in Toronto.